PRAISE FOR

REZOOM

"Nobody gives people the tools to transform their food from a health liability to a longevity asset like Susan Peirce Thompson. Bright Line Eating is truly life-saving for people who have struggled for years to unshackle themselves from the scourge of processed-food addiction."

— **Mark Hyman, M.D.**, *New York Times* best-selling author of *The Pegan Diet*

"I urge every doctor, therapist, health care practitioner, and most importantly every patient to read this book. *Rezoom* concisely and compassionately explains the emotional overlay that is a part of every person's interaction with food, and provides tools and skills that are game-changing for the occasional emotional eater clear to the raging food addict."

— **Wayne Dysinger, M.D.**, Board Chair, American Board of Lifestyle Medicine

"Therapists, social workers, eating disorders experts, and clinicians are unwittingly harming their patients when they spread the notion that food addiction is 'controversial.' The neuroscience is clear: food addiction is *real*. This book contains the best, scientifically based path to healing that I have seen."

— **Dr. Joy Jacobs, J.D., Ph.D.**, eating disorders specialist and clinical faculty in Psychiatry, University of California San Diego School of Medicine

"From the founding of Bright Line Eating, I have witnessed firsthand the astounding results for people in our community struggling with tenacious food addiction. They are healing their bodies and minds at extraordinary rates never before documented, while turning away from the toxic industrial processed food complex and healing our planet."

— **John Robbins**, best-selling author of *Diet for a New America* and President, Food Revolution Network

"If you suffer from a food addiction, this is the book that will set you free. It is brilliant, beautifully written, and desperately needed. Dr. Thompson's program not only works for weight loss, but it also works for optimal nutrition and health."

— **Brenda Davis, RD**, plant-based pioneer, speaker, and co-author of *Nourish*

"As a pediatrician with three decades of experience, the increasing rate of intractable obesity among my adolescent patients is nothing short of heart-breaking. I am so grateful to Dr. Susan Peirce Thompson and Bright Line Eating for this material contribution to saving me and the lives of my patients. She has changed my life and my practice, and she can change our world."

— **Judi A. Krogstad, M.D.**, Pediatric Medical Advisor, Fresno Metabolic and Bariatric Surgery Program

ALSO BY
SUSAN PEIRCE THOMPSON, Ph.D.

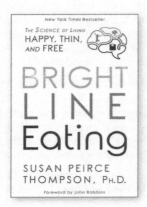
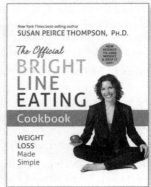

Both of the above are available at
your local bookstore, or may be ordered by visiting:

Hay House USA: www.hayhouse.com®
Hay House Australia: www.hayhouse.com.au
Hay House UK: www.hayhouse.co.uk
Hay House India: www.hayhouse.co.in

REZOOM

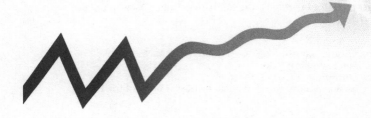

The Powerful Reframe to
END THE CRASH-AND-BURN CYCLE
of Food Addiction

SUSAN PEIRCE THOMPSON, Ph.D.

with Everett Considine

HAY
HOUSE

HAY HOUSE, INC.
Carlsbad, California • New York City
London • Sydney • New Delhi

Excerpt from *A Year with Rumi: Daily Readings* by Coleman Barks.
Copyright © 2006 by Coleman Barks. Used by permission of HarperCollins
Publishers.

Published in the United States by: Hay House, Inc.: www.hayhouse.com®
Published in Australia by: Hay House Australia Pty. Ltd.: www.hayhouse.com.au
Published in the United Kingdom by: Hay House UK, Ltd.: www.hayhouse.co.uk
Published in India by: Hay House Publishers India: www.hayhouse.co.in

Indexer: Joan Shapiro
Cover design: Julie Davison
Interior design: Bryn Starr Best
Brain scan illustration: Cinzia Damonte
All other graphs and illustrations: Angela Denby at Bright Line Eating

Cataloging-in-Publication Data is on file at the Library of Congress

Hardcover ISBN: 978-1-4019-5907-4
E-book ISBN: 978-1-4019-5908-1
Audiobook ISBN: 978-1-4019-5909-8

10 9 8 7 6 5 4 3 2 1
1st edition, December 2021

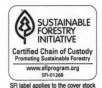

SUSTAINABLE
FORESTRY
INITIATIVE
Certified Chain of Custody
Promoting Sustainable Forestry
www.sfiprogram.org
SFI-01268
SFI label applies to the cover stock

Printed in the United States of America

For my Mastermind Group members, the Magnificent Mavens:
Cathy Cox, Linden Morris Delrio, and Marianne Marsh.
And for Christine (Chris) Gimeno Davis.

I learned to rezoom the hard way, and you were there.
And then some.

CONTENTS

CHAPTER 1

THE CYCLE OF RELAPSE

As of the writing of this book, I have been clean and sober from drugs and alcohol for 27 consecutive years. Prior to getting clean, I was a 20-year-old high school dropout addicted to crack cocaine and selling my body to stay high. After committing to recovery, I was able to complete my Ph.D. in brain and cognitive sciences, get married, and become the mother of three incredible kids. I know that everything I have in my life is dependent on one consistent, mandatory commitment: I *have* to stay clean and sober. But it isn't just a commitment. It is a practice. It is the application of a series of habits I have and choices I make every day that support my recovery.

I have also been abstinent from sugar and flour for 18 years. But not 100 percent perfectly. I estimate that for 94 percent of those days, my food recovery has been intact; some of the stretches have lasted for years and years. And then there were times when I was white-knuckling to string two abstinent days together. But my commitment to living free from the stranglehold of sugar and flour has allowed me to live the last 17 years in a slender body. To move through the world with energy and freedom. Then to lose that freedom and watch myself win it back. To return to a place where every day I am making life-affirming choices about how I care for myself with food.

I see myriad ways food recovery parallels drug and alcohol recovery, and important ways that they are qualitatively different. Frankly, food is uniquely wily and relapse more likely, for a host of reasons, so effective food recovery requires the dedication of a

Special Forces squadron commander. When I put the two experiences side by side and compare them, it can feel like, once it's solidly established, drug and alcohol recovery practically runs on autopilot. As someone who has experienced the gamut—hope-to-die drug addiction, decades of clean time, more relapse with food than I would wish on any breathing soul, years of consecutive abstinence from sugar and flour, decades of coaching people to achieve lasting recovery of all sorts, and years of teaching the neuroscience of food addiction in college courses—I offer this book as an instruction manual from a battle-tested expert in the field. I invite you to use it as a guidebook, keeping top of mind that food recovery isn't a one-and-done decision to lose weight and/or eat better. As with abstaining from drugs and alcohol, it's first a commitment and then a lifelong practice. And because your drug of choice must continue to be a part of your life multiple times a day, that practice involves a level of self-examination, grit, and vigilance unparalleled in the addiction-recovery landscape.

For the last seven years, I have been running a company that has helped thousands of people from over 100 countries make and sustain a commitment to lose weight and break free from food addiction. It is called Bright Line Eating (BLE), and when it comes to weight loss, it has long-term success rates unlike any other program out there. We have people in our community who have lived their entire lives addicted to sugar and flour, in various categories of obesity, who since coming to us are able to live in what I call Bright Bodies—ones that have reached their personal goal weight, enabling them to enjoy any activity, even just sitting still with themselves.

I created this program for them, not just because I had found a way to sustain my own Bright Body, which is an anomaly in the weight-loss annals, but because as a brain scientist I had hit upon ways to work *with* our brains, not against them, to accomplish seemingly impossible things.

But after several years, I noticed that while some people were able to embrace the tenets of Bright Line Eating, much as I had embraced the tenets of recovery from drugs and alcohol, others struggled.

The struggle, the cycle of success and failure, was its own animal. Meanwhile, as I was observing others' challenges, I was also going through my own. The gift of that confluence is that once I came out the other side, I had a new conception of how to manage a long-term food recovery journey that was unlike anything I had conceived of before—or seen offered to people struggling with food addiction.

What I learned is that if we reconceive relapse and learn to work *with* our cycles—in much the same way that Bright Line Eating works *with* our brains to release weight—instead of operating in a paradigm of "perfect" or "FUBAR," we begin to see recovery as a wave. Sometimes we are cresting high above the temptation to eat harmful foods, and sometimes we are skimming the bottom, but if we are honest with ourselves every day and gather that honesty as data, we can learn to coast, to surf our addiction without ever crashing on the rocks of relapse.

To help you do that, I am going to teach you how to rezoom. Whether you are an experienced Bright Lifer, have come to this book from a 12-Step food recovery program, or have been on your own journey with your food and weight, this book will give you three potent tools to end your relapse cycle. The first is the Rezoom Reframe, a powerful psychological shift that will fundamentally change the way you conceive of your journey. The second is the Rezoom System, the step-by-step guide to pouring your foundation strong so you stand on solid ground and have the tools to sustain it. And the third is a clinically proven psychological technique called Parts Work, which will ensure that every part of you is on board with your intention to live in your well-earned Bright Body, free of cravings and in alignment with the food you nourish yourself with every day.

Taken together, the three tools of rezooming compose an entire reframe in the domain of addiction, recovery, relapse, weight loss, and human behavior change. Learning to surf the rezoom wave without crashing requires learning the places where the rocks of relapse hide beneath the water. Now, of course people's experiences differ, but generally speaking there are a handful of common hiding spots that throw people off track. I've experienced them, some of them many times, and here's what I know: whether you feel like you're addicted to certain foods or not, whether you have 300 pounds to lose or 30, or zero, learning the most common places these rocks hide will be invaluable.

And nothing illustrates that like a story.

MY ADDICTION STORY

Addiction is a mysterious thing. I don't precisely know why I became addicted to the extent that I did. Certainly, I have addiction in my family. And the circumstances of my childhood were at least somewhat conducive; I was the only child of divorced parents who both worked hard to pay the bills, and I was alone a lot. I turned to food for entertainment, for comfort, for companionship.

Food became my first addiction, followed shortly by drugs. I started drinking and using in my hometown of San Francisco at age 14, and over the next six years, my drugs of choice got more and more dangerous and my life more and more chaotic. By an absolute miracle, I got clean and sober when I was 20. But my greatest addiction struggles were just beginning.

Several months into my recovery, I had a moment of clarity. I had enrolled in community college and was renting a little room in a shared house, and on one particular night I'd just come in from smoking a cigarette. It was now after 4 A.M., and whatever channel I'd been watching on TV had switched from programming to the wide, colorful vertical bars and the long, awful sound of "booooooop." I was sitting on the floor, surrounded by my binge foods—a pot of really cheap pasta with some kind of creamy cheese sauce, a near-empty bowl of raw cookie dough, an empty pint of ice cream, and a plate of mostly eaten English muffins slathered with butter and strawberry jam.

I was sitting there looking around, and the TV kept going "boooooop," and suddenly I had the deep awareness that *this is not sober behavior. I am using. This feels exactly like being in the crack house.*

But at that moment, I didn't know what to do about it.

A year later, after I had transferred from community college to UC Berkeley to major in cognitive science, someone finally tipped me off about what I could do. On their suggestion, I marched myself down to my first 12-Step food meeting. But people there weren't talking about addiction; they were talking about compulsive overeating. I was left to my own devices when it came to what to eat, what not to eat, and when and how to eat. I was told to "find a sponsor who has what you want," and maybe I wasn't willing, or maybe I never found the right sponsor, but the magic never happened.

I think of that period as eight years of yo-yoing, which is kind of like dieting, just with wonderfully supportive meetings to go to. My weight went up, my weight went down. But I could never reach the natural, healthy size that I am today, let alone stay there. The closest I got, for a brief moment, was about 20 pounds heavier than I am now. Overall, during those eight years, my weight went up. It peaked just above the "obese" marker on the BMI chart when I was about 26 years old.

More insidious, there was a lot of playing around with the food. I never got into a groove where I could move past my food and my weight as the focus du jour. It was always there. At various times I was reluctant to let go of all flour or all sweeteners, or I was eating yogurt with aspartame, or barbecue sauce, or I was stuck in a pattern of consuming half a dozen diet sodas a day and then awakening to the awareness that I was really addicted to them.

Without clear guidelines on precisely how to handle my food, I soldiered on, obsessed by food thoughts and struggling to manage my weight.

This period ended when I found a different 12-Step group that had broken away after recognizing the need to work a more rigorous program in order to achieve full recovery. People in this new group talked about food as an addiction. They were precise and prescriptive about what the addictive foods were and what to abstain from. In other words, they did the equivalent of defining the first drink so that members could get clear on what food recovery is.

I define food recovery (also known as abstinence, or playfully in Bright Line Eating, "squeaky-clean Bright Lines") as a way of eating that creates as much peace around food as the long-term sober alcoholic has around drinking. It is attained by eliminating sugar, flour, and any other foods that have hijacked the brain's reward center and putting boundaries around when and how much we eat.

By that time, the original 12-Step food group had formally disallowed consensus on food plans in their very bylaws. As a result, multiple other 12-step food programs cropped up because they concluded that they could not help anyone recover *without* being prescriptive. To them it would have been as preposterous as AA saying, "Well, choose whether you want to drink or not." And so a fundamental divide was born.

I feel like it's important to acknowledge, in a book about relapse, that the prescriptive program also worked in part by silencing the people who weren't having success in sticking to it. Relapse was still rampant, as it always is when true addiction is in play. But their approach to that reality was to not let anyone speak at a meeting unless they had maintained 90 days of continuous abstinence. It took a while to realize that only a small fraction of the people in the room at any given meeting were actually allowed to speak, share, and contribute, which, when I cottoned on, struck me as kind of horrifying and eerie.

However, under their auspices, I was abstinent, lost all my excess weight really fast, and was suddenly a size 4. This coincided with my move to Sydney, Australia, to do my postdoc in psychology at the University of New South Wales.

A few months after moving to Sydney, I found myself getting increasingly tired. It turned out that the congenital and not-yet-treated thyroid disease Hashimoto's hypothyroidism was creeping up on me. I was exhausted, and my recovery felt more and more like a rubber band that was stretching, stretching, stretching to the point where it had to break. It was clear to me that my abstinence was going to snap—and it was going to be bad.

When the moment came, I was in the open-air mall at Bondi Junction in Sydney. I went from food stall to food stall and ate and ate and ate. Then I threw it all up in a public bathroom and ate some more. This started the most painful, miserable, horrific time in my whole life as I watched myself grow from a size 4 to a size 24 in three months.

Early on in this period of relapse, my husband, David, informed me that we couldn't afford how I was eating, and he took away my credit and ATM cards. So, I radically simplified it. All I really needed was a sack of sugar that came in large discounted quantities, a sack of flour, and a big block of butter. And I would mash it all together in a metal bowl with a fork.

One hot summer day, I stumbled on an old receipt for some extra office supplies I deserved reimbursement for, and I got so excited that my hands started to shake. Right after the university bursar's office pushed the few bucks to me under the window, I immediately walked into the Randwick town square grocery store and got my sugar, flour, and butter so I could get that hit.

When people say, "Food can't be an addiction," I think, *Oh, you have no idea*.

MY VOW TO MYSELF

As the weeks and months rolled on, failing over and over again with every earnest attempt to stop eating addictively using the formula that had worked in the past, I just became more and more hopeless, despairing, and scared. One hot Sydney summer day, I was wearing my one muumuu dress. I had not showered in a while and I stank. I was walking back to my apartment with my big sack of sugar, my big sack of flour, and my big block of butter. My thighs were chafing together. Walking was laborious and painful.

On that walk I summoned up everything I had inside me and had a talk with myself in the sternest, most present, most soul-rattling tone I could muster. I said, "Susan, if you *ever* find yourself with ninety days of abstinence again, with that glorious peace and freedom, safe from the clutches of food, and the thought comes to eat off your plan, and that voice inside starts to convince you that it'll be delicious, that it'll be worth it, that you'll get away with it somehow, that you'll just get back on track later, that it won't be that bad, *you are promising yourself right now* that what you will do is physically go to the Golden Gate Bridge and jump off, not to die, but to let the smack of the cold water knock you back to your senses, because you must never, ever forget what this feels like. *This is the worst hell there is, and you must remember this moment."*

I was trapped in some kind of obscene, terrifying maze, where no matter what I did, I always seemed to be back in the same spot, eating enormous quantities of sugar and flour and not being able to stop. I had all the tools that used to work, but somehow they didn't work anymore. I couldn't conjure up the power, the force, to stop bingeing *and then stay stopped.*

During those three months, I burned through nine sponsors. And I remember wailing to one, "I'm doing everything. It's not working. It doesn't keep me from eating addictively the next day, or that day. Nothing stops me. I can battle mightily to stay abstinent for this one hour, but it's torture, and there's always some future Susan who will eat anyway, so why waste the effort now?"

She was very compassionate. She'd been through some relapse herself, and she said something to me I'll never forget for its simplicity and its wisdom and its comfort. She said, "Yeah, sometimes the addiction just needs to run its course."

So I started ad-libbing this prayer on my knees every day: "God, I'm in this food addiction hell, but I can imagine a day when I'm released again and experiencing ease and neutrality with my food. And God, just please hasten the day. Hasten the day that time comes. God, please *hasten the day."*

THE DAY ARRIVES

As a consequence of my addiction, I was floundering in my post-doc and feeling offtrack in life, so I hired a life coach. The first week we were working together, he gave me a homework assignment to complete before our next session and I balked at it. I agreed that the assignment had merit, but I said, "I just know I won't do it, because all I'm doing is eating."

"Okay, you've got to catch me up on what you mean."

I described what my life was like, what I was doing, and how I was struggling to get back on track with this program.

He asked, "Is this program really what you need?"

And I answered, "It's all there is, absolutely. What I need to do is stop eating addictively. I need to get back on my food plan. I've got to write down my food the night before, and commit it to a sponsor, and then eat only and exactly that."

And he said, "Well, Susan, you hired me, and if you can't do any work on anything in your life until you get this done, then this is the first thing. Your homework assignment for next week is to write down your food and eat only and exactly that. For seven consecutive days. And I'll talk to you next week."

I didn't think I could do it, but I agreed.

And it worked.

Somehow, I granted him authority in a way that I hadn't been able to grant a sponsor authority, and that commitment held me.

Chalk one up for finding the right accountability structure!

So began eight years of glory days with my food. I moved back to western New York, where I'd done my master's and Ph.D., became a psychology professor, and worked the 12 Steps over and over again. But there, too, I had a couple of "breaks," though I wouldn't call them breaks now—I would call them red flags and lessons.

The first was that artificial sweeteners were still allowed in that program (a huge loophole that serves no one—the science is clear on that). After I put a sugar-free syrup shot in my coffee at a café, the next day I went back and had another one, and then a stronger one, and suddenly I felt owned by artificial sweeteners. So I cut them out of my life. Lesson learned.

Then I was trying to balance my hormones by taking some supplements, like vitamin E and evening primrose oil in gelatin capsules. But instead of swallowing them, I was chewing them and feeling the oil explode in my mouth like a little firework, and it was just yummy. One day, I had my normal dose—and then a handful more. My sponsor said, "That's not taking supplements—that's a snack." And she put me back at Day 1.

I had eight years' adherence to my food plan, but the syrup and supplements show that food recovery can be a "both/and" situation. Yes, my food was clean and in its place, *and* there were times when the addiction would get reawakened and I would need to learn a helpful lesson and clean some things up.

That was my life all the way up until I decided to try to leave the 12-Step abstinence framework altogether.

A NECESSARY EXPERIMENT: A.K.A. PLAYING WITH FIRE

By the time my third daughter, Maya, was born, my twins were about to turn four, and I was concerned about giving them subtle, unhealthy messages from weighing and measuring my meals and eating differently than them. Also, I really wanted to model eating everything I was serving at the dinner table, including all the starch kids need.

At that point, after eight years of sanity and stability, I felt healed and whole. I genuinely didn't believe that I could ever, would ever, hurt myself with food again. I thought that, with enough support and the right honest motivations, I would successfully be able to reintroduce all foods back into my life—including foods made of sugar and flour. The permission-based approach I wanted to try is called competent eating, described very well by Ellyn Satter in her *Feeding with Love and Good Sense* book series. You get to eat whatever you want, at mealtime, until you feel absolutely satisfied. But while I found that sometimes my natural "stopping place" was a very moderate amount of food, at other times I could eat eight sugar cookies the size of a medium dinner plate and very calmly reason, *No, I don't think I'm satisfied yet. I think I really want one more.* And I would keep going.

Of course, my weight started to creep up. I had expected that and thought I was prepared to accept it. But when size 4 became size 6 and threatened to keep climbing, I had to ask myself how many new wardrobes of clothes I was willing to buy in service of this experiment. The answer was none. Therefore, I had to start putting boundaries around my eating. That put me into a whole new universe because in the Competent Eating/Intuitive Eating world, there could be no such boundaries. Full permission was a must.

So I abandoned the full permission idea and tried other approaches . . . and my life got more and more unmanageable. My *thinking* got more and more unmanageable. I started to feel, once again, like a hamster on a wheel. Suddenly I had a crappy new full-time job managing my food and weight, and I didn't want it.

But I think the urge to try this experiment, after some months or years of food recovery, is something that nearly every recovering food addict is going to have. Because experiencing the peace, ease, and relative normalcy of successful food recovery is very much like the person with schizophrenia who forgets that it's the medicine they're taking that is helping them be well.

They say insanity is doing the same thing over and over again and expecting different results. I would add that insanity is finding what really works and then deciding to stop doing it.

Two and a half months after the Competent Eating experiment began, I went back to the 12-Step program, the rigid one that worked. At that point I was pretty desperate again. I cried. I couldn't stop eating ice cream. I felt out of control and really scared. But once I surrendered the addictive foods and got back on a simple food plan, I was abstinent again for another three years. Which brings us to the birth of Bright Line Eating.

BRIGHT LINES

It was impossible to be living in my right-sized body, surrounded by friends and family I cared about who were struggling with their weight, and not feel the need for a broader, more workable version of the doctrinaire 12-Step program I was in. When I taught my Psychology of Eating course, most of my college students needed some help with their food and their weight, yet rarely did any of them come and check out the program. As a mother of young children, I knew it was too exacting with its requirements, for example, to attend three 90-minute meetings a week . . . forever. So when I heard, "Write a book called Bright Line Eating," during my regular meditation one dark, winter morning, I guess I was ready. I started working toward getting a Bright Line Eating book published and learned pretty quickly that I needed to build an audience first. So I launched the Bright Line Eating email list, and before long it mushroomed into a worldwide movement.

During that first year, I was the Assistant Chair of the Psychology department while teaching four or five college courses each semester. I was still in that 12-Step program for food addiction and doing 20 to 30 hours of volunteer work a week for that organization in various capacities. My daughters were still little, and I was making dinner every night for the family and working with my husband to get the kiddos through bath time and story time and bedtime. *And* I also grew Bright Line Eating to the point where it was serving thousands of people in 90 countries around the world. I was so passionate about the work that somehow I just squeezed it all in. Honestly, I don't know how.

For that first year, I kept my Lines Bright amidst the unspeakable overload and intensity and excitement that my life had become. And then I was at a baby shower, and I broke my Lines. There were platters of food out, which is a tricky situation, and the way to navigate it is to put what you're going to eat on your plate and be done.

But I didn't do that. I just kept going back to the platters and eating cheese and salami, cheese and salami. There was a point where I noticed that I was eating too much, and I kept going. I always say, "When you become aware, you become responsible." At that moment, I didn't want to be responsible—I just wanted to eat. And I kept going.

After eating my fill, I went out to the car and sat there for a long time before driving home. I thought back to Sydney, how my universe had altered completely and profoundly with that first addictive bite. Was I now back on that horrific roller coaster that would take me into the depths of a living hell?

To fight against that, I tried to make meaning out of what had just happened, because my life was not the same as it had been when I lived in Sydney. I was now a very public figure representing a new way of eating, and every week I went on camera sharing my experience, my perspective, and my scientific knowledge.

At that time I only had one template for a relapse: this is the end of the world as you know it. But there was a huge difference this time. I could *not* gain weight because my identity as someone who needed to share a message of recovery from food addiction through Bright Lines was so deep and so strong. And I knew that I couldn't be credible as the Bright Line Eating spokesperson if I gained a bunch of weight. So I was forced to rethink relapse.

Right up front, I had to grapple with the framework I had internalized: that anyone who has recently taken an addictive bite of food clearly knows nothing about food recovery and has to be silent. Impostor syndrome is hardly uncommon, but boy, was it especially strong in me at that juncture.

I started down a radical new path when, a short while later, I decided to be public about the fact that I was struggling with my food and released a video called *The Morning After a Binge*. The surge of positive, reassuring comments beneath that video felt like cold running water on burned skin. What surprised me most was that people felt my video had *helped them*. It burst the bubble of isolation and shame they were living in and made them more apt to follow, not less. Thus, I encouraged a culture in Bright Line Eating to invite and elevate the voice of the Rezoomer, while still wholeheartedly celebrating long stretches of unbroken Bright Lines.

The next set of years was a maelstrom. I wish I could say that I had one or two breaks and stayed Bright from then on, but alas, it took me quite a while to learn to stay consecutively Bright again amidst the intensity that had become my new life. Once the option to eat over stress was back on the table, the pernicious urgency of my food addiction, bumping up against the necessity to not eat addictively in order to maintain my role as the leader of Bright Line Eating on camera, created an accelerated learning environment—a pressurized laboratory. And within four years, I got more experience in breaking and rezooming than I might have gotten over four decades if there hadn't been so much pressure exerted by those two forces.

Whenever I broke, I was honest about it in the Bright Line Eating community. The love and compassion that flowed in allowed me to watch my journey and extract its lessons. And as the cycles of breaking and rezooming continued, the nature of the cycles changed.

First, I learned to remain calm and gentle. When a break happened, I'd just immediately orient myself toward some very simple actions to correct the situation with a guiding voice inside that said, *This is not an emergency. This happens sometimes, and we know exactly how to address it.*

Then the breaks became spread so far apart that I was really living Bright for the most part.

And then the breaks stopped.

THE INTERVENTIONS

The three elements that supported me in making this shift are the focus of this book. And they inextricably work hand in hand. The first is the Rezoom Reframe, which I will teach you in Chapter 4. This shift will enable you to approach your breaks like a compassionate scientist, gathering data to continually strengthen your program. The second is a set of behavioral interventions I'm going to teach you that I call the Rezoom System. They are designed to up-level your choices around your food (Chapter 5), your actions (Chapter 6), and your support (Chapter 7) so your recovery stays humming, with your food and your weight handled, so you can focus on life.

However, if those are the only tools you have, in my experience, the problem is you won't use them. At least not consistently. Inner resistance will crop up and create some form of self-sabotage. That's where the third element comes in. At the end of each chapter, you will be introduced to a remarkably effective way to clear your inner resistance so you can actually follow through on living Bright.

Your guide for these sections is Everett Considine, an expert in Parts Work, which is a therapeutic approach based on something called Internal Family Systems (IFS). After I ate all that salami and cheese at the baby shower, I reached out to Everett for help. He taught me how to access the part of me who wanted to binge and gave me the tools to escape the clutches of those cravings. And because Parts Work is particularly good at unlocking deep self-compassion, he helped me reorient toward my breaks in a loving way.

What we're going to be covering in these Parts Work sections is a fuller exposition on what, in my first book, *Bright Line Eating*, I simply referred to as the Saboteur—the whisper that encourages us to eat addictively, but in our own voice. This was a beginner's concept that implicitly set up the Saboteur as a combatant, a thing to be battled and overcome. But once you're a little way into your journey, there is a lot more healing and a lot more self-compassion available through diving in and conceiving of the Saboteur in a richer and more nuanced way.

So whether you are an experienced Bright Lifer, someone coming to this book through a 12-Step program, or even someone who has never done any formal food recovery but is just getting curious about their relationship with food and whether it might be addictive to some degree, there will be valuable information for you in these pages. Even if you feel your struggles with food are minor and peripheral or you only sometimes notice that you're not eating in alignment with your values and intentions for yourself, read on. The Rezoom Reframe is likely to forever change your sense of agency as you navigate your relationship with food.

But this book is especially for you if you're "in the ditch"— our phrase in Bright Line Eating for the hellish Groundhog Day of bingeing and struggling to stop bingeing that had me trapped in Sydney. Just as the Lorax says, "I am the Lorax. I speak for the trees," I speak for the people who suffer with profound, overwhelming obsession and compulsion with food. Because the suffering is great. My cherished goal is to help, serve, and connect with those who feel beyond help. Beyond.

My goal is to provide you comfort, deep empathy borne of understanding, and, most importantly, a road map out.

As Rumi says:

> *There is a secret medicine*
> *given only to those who hurt so hard*
> *they can't hope.*

I pray that, within these pages, you will find that medicine.

I will show you what to do to end the painful crash-and-burn cycles and convert them into the smooth, continuous flow that results in a recovered body and mind. Everett will help you get your whole self on board so you'll actually do it.

By combining the external actions with the inner work, you will have an unbeatable approach to attaining and then, with a modicum of daily effort, maintaining your Bright Transformation—without the anguish of relapse.

It's time to dive in.

PARTS WORK INTRODUCTION

Welcome to Parts Work, where we address getting our whole psyche aligned with our weight-loss journey. Parts Work is relatively simple and intuitive. You can access it best by reflecting back on your own experience.

Have you ever felt like there is some part of you that seems to have a separate agenda? A part that wants to eat off your plan or engage in behaviors that you know will undermine your program? Or do you feel you have a part that is amazing at managing your food—until it isn't—and then "someone else" takes over and eats with abandon? In working with thousands of people recovering from food addiction, we can say with assurance that these are all common experiences. In these end-of-chapter sections, we will give you the tools to meet, befriend, and integrate these parts, so that every component of your psyche—and yes, we all have components to our psyche—is supporting your healing journey.

The "parts" perspective has a long and esteemed history. Socrates, Aristotle, Plato, Nietzsche, Freud, and Jung all talked about the human psyche having parts. But the modern-day version of Parts Work that we are focused on in this book began in the 1980s when psychologist and academic Richard Schwartz, Ph.D., was working with bulimic patients and noticed that many of them talked about having different parts of themselves. They said they had a part that would binge. They had a part that would purge. They had a part that could control going long stretches without doing either.

Curious, he started helping his patients get to know these parts better. What he found was that he could actually ask them to dialogue with the parts, and his patients could relate whole conversations between these parts of themselves. He learned that the parts existed in relationship to one another and that there was actually frequent tension among the parts because each part had a different agenda. He discovered that a patient could recognize when a specific part was present. And Schwartz could prompt the patient to ask that part to step aside, and the angry—or sad, or vindictive, or betrayed—part would actually comply.

What he evolved over time is now known as the Internal Family Systems (IFS) model of the psyche, named as such because he came to see our parts, or subpersonalities, as interacting with each other in ways similar to a family—with both cooperation and conflict.

Internal Family Systems therapy is widely used to treat trauma, anxiety, depression, eating disorders, addiction, and other behavioral problems. It is an incredibly powerful modality to support rapid changes in unwanted behaviors.

Below is an introduction to how IFS works. At the end of each subsequent chapter, we will cover a common part that people encounter on their rezoom journeys, so you can begin to think about the role your parts may have played in relapse in the past. In Appendix B, you will find quizzes and an inventory so you can begin to engage with any parts you identified.

As you dig into this work, you might find some components triggering, especially if you have a history of complex trauma. Focusing on our parts can take us quickly to the root of a matter, and for some, that can cause a little dysregulation. Go gently and slowly and reach out for support if you need it. It takes courage to do our "inner work," but we get *so* many rewards when we do.

Authentic Self

At the center of the IFS model of the psyche is the Authentic Self, with a capital S. Schwartz discovered in his clinical work that we *all* have an Authentic Self, a calm, clear center underneath the storm of our parts. We have eight qualities when we are in Authentic Self, and we call them the "8 Cs": calm, confidence, curiosity, creativity, clarity, courage, compassion, and connectedness. In this work, we are trying to live more deeply and completely from a place of our Authentic Self. As you start to explore your inner system of parts, you will quickly begin to notice when you are operating from your Authentic Self versus when you are operating from a wounded or protective part.

Our Parts

Our parts primarily fall into two categories: wounded parts and protective parts. Wounded parts often (but certainly not always) stem from childhood, when we were mistreated or abused, or suffered pain, difficulty, or loss. Our protective parts take on the job of looking after our wounded parts, while also keeping them out of view. The category of protective parts breaks down further into Managers and Firefighters.

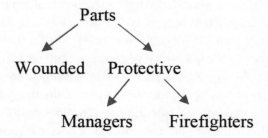

The Manager's self-appointed job is to be our *proactive* protector, to help us live our life in such a way that we don't experience pain. I'm sure you can see the problem with that right up front. Pain is a natural part of life, and sadness and anger are essential core emotions. Parts that have the thankless job of trying to keep us from those emotions are going to wreak a lot of havoc in trying to accomplish the impossible.

To illustrate this, let's imagine a young woman whose overly critical mother always told her that she didn't measure up and now has a wounded part that feels deficient. A

Manager then develops and decides: *To not feel deficient, I am going to excel! I'm going to work harder than everyone else, and I'll prove to my mom that I'm worth something.*

The young woman goes to an amazing school and gets an advanced degree and works really hard to get repeatedly promoted. And all of this is being driven by the Manager, which never wants her to feel that deficiency. But when she makes a mistake at work, or gets some criticism on a 360 review, or someone swipes left on her, or she goes home to see her mom, that deficiency gets triggered because in her wounded part's eyes, she's afraid she can never be good enough. The Manager part collapses in exhaustion and defeat.

What might happen next is that a reactive protector, a Firefighter, might swoop in to numb the pain, and suddenly she wants to drink or smoke or eat or do something so as to not feel the triggered wound. That's what Firefighter parts do, because they are our *reactive* protectors—they come in after we've been wounded. They're the ones calling the shots over Thanksgiving weekend when grown adults back with their families are smoking on their roofs, hitting their hometown bars, or eating a bunch of candy in their cars. The more moderate Firefighter escapes are television, web surfing, computer games, shopping, overeating, caffeine, cigarettes, cocktails, sleeping, sex, dieting, prescription drugs, exercising, flirting, lying, anger, sarcasm, gambling, car racing, fantasizing, and procrastination.

Some of the extreme Firefighter manifestations are bingeing and purging, anorexia, suicidal ideation, stealing, shoplifting, panic attacks, running away, cutting, sexual compulsivity, abuse of alcohol and drugs, rage, emotional abuse, violence, sexual abuse, and murder.

Please know that if anything on that list was triggering for you, we *all* have Managers, and we *all* have Firefighters. There's nothing wrong with you for having them. The work now is helping parts that have taken on extreme roles to come back into balance in our lives. In IFS, we are not trying to get rid of parts; we are trying to bring them back into balance.

In addition, it is essential to always remember that *our parts are trying to help us*. For that reason, we must always hold them in a place of curiosity and compassion, even when we discover a part that may have caused some real damage in our life.

Frequently our parts develop as coping strategies in childhood, so they have the hallmarks of a child's developing brain, such as limited perspective, absolutism, inflexibility, or an abundance of fear. If you have a beloved child in your life, think of how they handle confrontation or challenge ("No, I didn't!" "It's mine!" "I don't want to _____, it's scary!"), and extend to yourself and your parts the same patience, humor, and love that you extend to them.

The exciting work begins when you identify a part of yourself that needs some love and attention, some compassion and patience, and then experience the shift that happens when you give that gift to yourself, unlocking a new peace around your food and your recovery that you never thought possible. Through the Parts Work sections at the end of each chapter, we will hold your hand on that journey.

CHAPTER 2

FOOD ADDICTION IS REAL

Many years ago, I knew a man named Lonnie. Like me, he was a recovering drug addict. He'd been clean from heroin for over 30 years and was a shining example of what recovery can do in a person's life. He was stable, grounded, funny, educated, magnanimous, popular, and actively in service to his community. He had a beautiful relationship with his wife and cherished his young daughter above all else. Everybody loved Lonnie.

And Lonnie was a food addict. He was massively overweight and diagnosed with cellulitis, high blood pressure, and type 2 diabetes, and over the following three years, I kept getting reports of how badly he was deteriorating. He tried the normal routes of diet and exercise, but with little sustainable success. He kept returning to high-sugar foods. A friend of mine, a recovering drug addict who was also actively in recovery for his own food addiction, talked with Lonnie and said, "Hey, man, you're a food addict. This is serious. You've got to change how you're eating. If you don't confront this, it will kill you."

But for all his decades of work in recovery, Lonnie couldn't— or wouldn't—apply what had worked for him with drugs, alcohol, cigarettes, and even gambling, to food. Finally, he said to our mutual friend, "I'm gonna let the food take me."

Before long, he couldn't see well enough to leave the house and he couldn't walk anymore.

And then he died.

With decades of recovery from drug addiction under his belt, he died of food addiction.

While Lonnie's story is extreme, it's not that uncommon. Many, many people come into Bright Line Eating having been told by their doctors that they are eating themselves to death, whether from diabetes, heart disease, or any number of other diseases and conditions. The excess weight, calories, and sugar are putting an unsustainable strain on their bodies.

And even if they haven't reached that point in their medical journey, many people still have a relationship with food that qualifies as addictive. Which is not surprising. Corporations have invested billions over the last few decades engineering modern "food" to be as addictive as possible, and it's working.

But here's the thing: not every obese person is a food addict, and not every food addict is obese. Surprisingly, food addiction is less correlated with weight than you might think. In Bright Line Eating, we use a Food Addiction Susceptibility Scale that goes from 1 to 10, with 10 being high. You can get your score at FoodAddictionQuiz.com. It's only five questions and designed to reveal how strongly your brain gets pulled in by addictive foods.

If your score is between 1 and 3, you are at the low end of the scale. This means your body gives you reliable signals about when to stop eating. You likely never binge, aren't plagued by strong food cravings, and tend to be thinking about your *life* rather than your weight or what you feel like eating next. Our data show that 32 percent of people with a BMI in the overweight range are actually low on the Susceptibility Scale, as are 19 percent of people with obesity and 12 percent of people with severe obesity.[1] Typically, these are people who just need to follow the Bright Line Eating food plan for a bit to get the weight off and then focus on practicing the habits we will cover in Chapter 6.

A score of 4 to 7 is in the midrange, which may mean you think of yourself as having some amount of challenge with food. How much probably depends on whether you're overweight and whether or not you have health issues. But you're no stranger to cravings and likely spend more time than you'd prefer thinking about your food and your weight. And alas, once you start eating, there's no guarantee that you'll stop at a place you feel good about.

Forty-three percent of people who are overweight are in the mid-range on the Susceptibility Scale, as are 48 percent of people with obesity and 32 percent of people with severe obesity. For people in the midrange, I strongly advocate staying strict at first while the brain heals and then experimenting with what allows you to stay free. There's no CliffsNotes I can give you on which Bright Lines you'll be able to flex and how, because people *differ* in what gives them peace. But be conservative, especially if you're coming from bigger numbers on the bathroom scale. The brain tends to want to coax people back up to their former high weight, and the hormonal shifts it creates to ensure that happens can push people higher on the Susceptibility Scale. But no worries. Once you live in a Bright Body with peace and freedom around food, you won't let yourself live any other way for long.

If you've scored an 8 or above, you're highly susceptible to food addiction and you've probably struggled with your eating and/or your weight for years, if not decades. The signals that tell other people to stop eating just don't work for you. Depending on how high your score is, you may have a horrific history of binge-ing. You may or may not have an eating disorder (or a history of one). But almost for sure, you're spending more time think-ing about what you've eaten or not eaten, what you want to eat next, and what you weigh or wish you weighed than feels sane or appropriate.

On the Susceptibility Scale, I am a perfect 10. In fact, to quote Spinal Tap, I probably go to 11. Here's the simple truth I've dis-covered after years and years of trying everything under the sun: plans of moderation and intuitive eating *do not* work for people who are high on the Susceptibility Scale because bona fide addic-tion is in play.

We're going to examine what exactly that means now.

THE EVOLVING SCIENTIFIC CONVERSATION

Shockingly, with obesity raging as a global pandemic despite a multibillion-dollar diet industry, the construct of food addiction is still highly controversial in the scientific literature.[2] The history behind the controversy goes back to the origins of eating disorder treatment, which burgeoned in the 1970s with the diagnoses of bulimia nervosa and anorexia nervosa. The foundational tenet of treating those disorders became *no food rules*. To achieve full recovery, a patient must be willing to eat all foods in moderation because that is what "normal" eating looks like.

Within this framework, the notion of food addiction is extremely problematic because as soon as you start talking about addiction, in the very next breath you ask, "What would treatment look like?" And boom, some sort of abstinence has to come into the mix. Meaning food rules, which are considered triggering, restrictive, and counterproductive. Still today, professional education in the domain of eating disorder treatment usually takes the eat-everything-in-moderation approach.

Dr. Joy Jacobs is an eating disorder specialist with a Ph.D. in clinical psychology. She is clinical faculty of psychiatry at the University of California San Diego and has an overflowing practice treating patients with every form of eating disorder. When she first started her practice 16 years ago, there was not a single mainstream eating disorder treatment center that would let patients be vegetarian, let alone vegan. No matter the reason. Patients with ethical objections, or for whom meat causes constipation, would be required to eat chicken, beef, or perhaps pork for dinner. Dr. Jacobs's specialized and rigorous training took place in settings that required patients in recovery to eat cookies, cake, doughnuts, and other sugary foods, often several times per day. Patients who refused were considered highly eating-disordered and would have privileges revoked for such refusal in the token economies often utilized in inpatient treatment settings. Over the years, she noticed it wasn't working very well. "Every time some of my patients would eat a cookie or other sugary food, they'd be off to the races again. I started to think, maybe they really shouldn't be required to eat those foods. Maybe moderate consumption of those foods is not possible or advisable for these patients."

Interestingly, we now know that about half of individuals with an eating disorder also meet the criteria for food addiction. Among patients with bulimia nervosa, it's even higher, ranging from 81.5 percent all the way up to 100 percent. But once the bulimia is in remission, the rate of food addiction goes down to 30 percent.[3]

By the turn of the 21st century, researchers were starting to look at compulsive eating behavior in a new way. More and more studies were showing the similar neurological effects of processed foods and drugs of abuse on the reward pathways in the brain. In 2007, Yale University's Rudd Center for Food Policy and Obesity hosted 40 experts from around the world to discuss food as an addiction. "Everything changes if food is found to have addictive properties, especially the legal and legislative landscape around marketing foods to children," said Dr. Kelly Brownell, then director of the center. "People often use the language of addiction to explain their relationship with food cravings, withdrawal, irresistible impulses—it is all there."[4]

One of the many great things that emerged from that meeting was the development in 2009 of the Yale Food Addiction Scale, which is similar to the Susceptibility Scale. Using their metric, they have consistently found that 19.9 percent of the general population has food addiction, which is essentially the same percentage as scores 9 and 10 on our instrument.[5]

THE DIAGNOSIS OF FOOD ADDICTION

The American Psychiatric Association is strangely touchy when it comes to the word *addiction*, which is bizarre because we're so comfortable with that term everywhere else. The media is comfortable with it. Professors are comfortable with it. Clinicians and people who deliver frontline treatment use the term *addiction* all the time. But the official diagnosis in the *DSM-5*, the American Psychiatric Association's *Diagnostic and Statistical Manual of Mental*

Disorders, is Substance Use Disorder. Within this framework, even if you're shooting heroin every day, you're not a heroin addict—you have a Heroin Use Disorder. Substance Use Disorders come in a bunch of other categories too, many of them familiar to us all: alcohol, caffeine, cannabis, hallucinogens, inhalants, opioids, stimulants, sedatives, tobacco, and other/unknown.

Is food addiction then called Food Use Disorder? The answer is no (and not because that terminology would be ridiculous, given that regular "food use" is a requirement for being alive). Food and eating aren't mentioned in the Substance Use Disorder section at all. The only behavioral disorder the *DSM-5* recognizes is gambling disorder. Sex, exercise, and shopping are mentioned in passing but not included because "currently there is insufficient peer-reviewed evidence to establish these behaviors as mental disorders."[6] The addictive aspects of food and eating are simply ignored altogether. Perhaps there's even less peer-reviewed evidence to establish addictive eating as a legitimate disorder than, say, addictive shopping or addictive exercising, but that's honestly hard to believe. I have two college textbooks on my desk—*Processed Food Addiction: Foundations, Assessment, and Recovery* and *Compulsive Eating Behavior and Food Addiction: Emerging Pathological Constructs*—each of which cites hundreds and hundreds of peer-reviewed studies.

So should processed foods be given the same status as caffeine, alcohol, heroin, cannabis, and all the rest? Well, there are 11 criteria for thoughts and behaviors that qualify someone for a Substance Use Disorder in the *DSM-5*.[7] Let's see how food stacks up.

1) Unintended use. Consuming a substance in greater amounts or over longer periods of time than intended. Are there people who routinely eat more than they intended, or maybe keep eating longer than they intended? I think we can all wholeheartedly agree that food meets this criterion and then some.

It could run the gamut, of course. From confronting a buffet table and intending to have a little but suddenly having an overflowing plate, to someone who thinks they're going to just have a taste of their roommate's ice cream, and before they know it, they've finished the whole thing, which now necessitates a run to the convenience store at 1:00 in the morning to replace the pint before their roommate gets back. Or maybe you bought groceries, intending them to be for someone else, for a party, or to last a whole week, and before you know it, it's all eaten, and you've got to go get more. Whether it's a little unintended use or a whole lot, that feeling of losing control over how much you're eating is one of the hallmarks of food addiction.

2) **Failure to cut back.** This criterion involves having a persistent desire to decrease or limit your use of the substance, with many unsuccessful attempts to keep it in check. The whole diet industry is based on this. Research shows that about *half of Americans* are on a diet at any given moment, and among that half, the average person makes four or five new attempts each year.[8]

3) **Time spent.** This means spending a significant amount of time acquiring, using, or recovering from a substance. Eighteen years ago, on the first day that I intended to eat only three meals and put my food on a digital food scale, I remember weighing my breakfast and then being overcome by a yawning chasm between that moment and lunchtime. I was so used to eating my way through time that the thought of not eating again until lunch terrified me, and I really hadn't been aware until then of how much time I was spending acquiring food, eating, and then lying on the couch recovering from eating. A lot of people in Bright Line Eating are pretty stunned by how much time is freed up.

4) **Cravings.** Craving the substance or having a strong urge to use it is another slam dunk. We all know that certain foods produce intense cravings (at least in most people), and food manufacturers know it too. Craveability is a central feature of myriad food commercials—melting cheese and swirling chocolate abound.

A quick story on the power of cravings. One time when I was in my early 20s and the holidays came around, my then-boyfriend and I drove across the border into Canada to visit his family. On the way back along the thruway, I saw a sign for Mrs. Fields Cookies.

I'm from California. Mrs. Fields is from California. But I had not seen one of those stores since I'd moved to western New York. I didn't say anything. We just drove on. It took another hour of driving for him to drop me off at my apartment. I said, "Bye," and waited for him to leave. Then I got in *my* car and drove all the way back. Only now it was closed. So then I drove all the way home again, but first I went to the grocery store because I had already obviously planned a binge.

Being willing to go out of your way to get a particular food, to make the extra trip for the ingredient you just *have* to have, to go out in a snowstorm to get the takeout—these are cravings. They pull us beyond reason.

5) Failure to fulfill roles. This means being unable to fulfill obligations at work, school, or home due to use of a substance. When I was on the merry-go-round with food, with recovery and relapse, recovery and relapse, every time I went back into the food, I could not function as a wife and a mother. I would check out almost completely, and at the worst times.

When my husband and I took our kids on a long-awaited Disney cruise, a couple of days in, I ate some sugar. Suddenly I was incapable of showing up to spend time with my family. I stayed away from everyone—in our cabin or on the adults-only deck—hiding and just eating, eating, eating. I was useless; I could not fulfill my role, especially as a mother. I missed all the fun, and it was extremely painful for me, for my husband, for my kids. I tried to hide it to some degree from the kids, but I don't know how well I did.

6) Interpersonal problems. This means continually using a substance despite its effects causing or exacerbating persistent or recurrent social or interpersonal problems. For example, a few years ago I joined a mastermind group of online entrepreneurs and showed up on the first evening at a socializing event. Immediately, this guy beelines over to me and says, "I know who you are, and I need to talk to you." He wasn't morbidly obese, but he was a big guy, and he knew he had a major problem with food. He wanted to learn more about it, and he was wondering if I could help.

At some point during that evening, his live-in girlfriend joined us. She had all the signs of a deeply scarred and war-weary codependent partner. She got choked up often. Her facial expressions showed occasional flashes of desperation. Her eyes were pleading. She wanted to convey to me the painful extremes he went through in multiple areas of his life due to his continued dysfunctional relationship with food and what it was like for her to try to help him. It was a huge issue in their relationship and a huge injury to her. Every day, month, year that his food addiction raged on, she was being inadvertently harmed. It can be so hard when we are in the food to think about how it is affecting those around us, but it is, I can assure you.

7) Giving up or reducing social, occupational, or recreational activities due to substance use. Frequently when people come to Bright Line Eating, their lives have gotten very small. They don't fly because the seats are too small. They can't roll on the floor with their grandkids, or ride a bike, or play golf. Some report feeling isolated because they feel stigmatized in public. Whether it's shame or physical discomfort, the end result is the same. Their eating has come between them and the life they imagined for themselves.

8) Hazardous use. I have a friend who worked in her 20s as a shuttle driver of adults with deafness and cognitive disabilities. She had blood sugar issues and was severely addicted to sugar. During her long days of shuttling folks to their jobs, she would binge on sugar, and the insulin spikes and blood sugar crashes would make her so tired she would nod off at the wheel. She knew she was endangering the lives of her passengers, and she kept promising herself that she wouldn't eat sugar on the job. But she just couldn't stop. That's hazardous use.

9) Continually using a substance despite physical or psychological problems that are caused or made worse by the substance. This is another obvious one when you think of the impact of food on health. Sixty-three percent of people in America are dying in pain and prematurely from diseases that we know are food and lifestyle related.[9] And after the diagnosis of heart disease or type 2 diabetes, when there's still the potential for disease remission or even complete reversal if the right diet is adopted, people just don't. Like Lonnie, whose story opened this chapter, they continue to use the food they want or think they need despite the physical problems that are being made worse by the substance.

10) Tolerance. This means needing a substantially higher dose of the substance to achieve the desired effect or experiencing a substantially reduced effect of the substance when the usual dose is consumed. Back in 2015 and 2016, the few times when my addictive eating went on beyond a couple of days, I noticed I would start to need so much more sugar and flour that I would essentially stop eating all other foods. I just had no room, even though I love salad. Over a few days, I would build such a rapid tolerance to sugar and flour that it would end up being my whole diet.

11) Withdrawal. We see this in our community, and I warn readers of my first book, *Bright Line Eating*, to expect it. Typically, people starting Bright Line Eating experience uncomfortable withdrawal symptoms when they first stop consuming sugar and flour, including muscle aches, nausea, headache, and fatigue.

Those are the 11 criteria.

Now I'm going to share something stunning. *All you need to qualify for a diagnosis of Substance Use Disorder is 2 out of those 11.* That's it. Two. That's for a mild case. Moderate would be 4 or 5 symptoms, and the most severe classification only requires 6 of those 11 symptoms. This blows my mind. You don't need all of them, or even close to all of them. All you need to have for the most severe classification is 6 of those symptoms.

The bottom line is that millions of people are hurting themselves with addictive eating, and they're trying to stop but they can't. The *DSM-5* itself says, "The essential feature of a substance use disorder is . . . that the individual continues using the substance despite significant substance-related problems."[10] Every year in the United States, 130,000 people have a leg amputated due to uncontrolled diabetes.[11] And they still can't stop eating addictively, so 55 percent of them will have their *second leg* amputated within two years.[12] If that isn't continuing to use despite significant substance-related problems, I don't know what is.

THE NEUROSCIENCE OF FOOD ADDICTION

Counselors, clinicians, and social workers who have been trained in a "no food rules" paradigm for treating eating disorders might consider the construct of food addiction controversial. But I'll tell you who doesn't: neuroscientists, addiction specialists, and addiction researchers, who recognize that food has the potential to impact the brain the same way as other addictive substances and behaviors. They recognize that the brains of food addicts have the same characteristic features as other addicted brains, not just in one pathway but in multiple areas.

In fact, the 2018 review article "What Is the Evidence for 'Food Addiction'? A Systematic Review"[13] looked at every paper on the construct of food addiction that was both quantitative and peer-reviewed and found studies supporting every characteristic of addiction in relation to food, with the largest number of studies examining the brain reward dysfunction that underlies food addiction.

In my first book, *Bright Line Eating*, my Food Freedom video series, and countless webinars, I have described that science in simple terms. Addictive foods flood the nucleus accumbens in the reward center of the brain with excess dopamine, and over time those dopamine receptors downregulate. They become less numerous, less responsive. As this process takes root, continued use, or increased use, is necessary to feel just a baseline level of "okayness."

Here's a figure of a PET scan showing what addictive eating does to the brain.

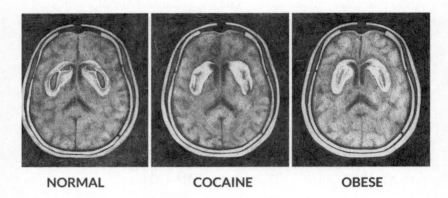

NORMAL   COCAINE   OBESE

On the left is a normal brain showing a healthy dopamine response. In the middle, the dopamine receptors in the nucleus accumbens have been blown out with repeated cocaine use. But notice that the brain of the obese subject shows the same blunted and muted dopamine response as the cocaine-addicted brain. This is what happens when you've overeaten foods laden with sugar and flour for years and years and years. A neuroscientist looking at the neurological changes associated with excess food consumption would say, "There's the food addiction right there." It's not confusing.

It turns out that prolonged exposure to addictive foods isn't just linked with dopamine downregulation but with serotonin downregulation, endocannabinoid downregulation, and endogenous opioid receptor downregulation as well. The net result is a negative mood and a general sense of malaise and discomfort. Unless, of course, you combat it with another trip to the kitchen, convenience store, or drive-thru. A bout of addictive eating will flood the brain with exactly the cocktail of neurotransmitters it needs to feel that all's right with the world again—and each of those pathways will downregulate yet a tiny bit more.

In addition to neurotransmitter downregulation, the hallmark of addiction in the brain, two additional lines of research show changes in the brain associated with food addiction, both of which are present with drug addiction. The first is called cue reactivity, and the second is cognitive impairment.

Cue reactivity is a heightened response in the reward centers of the brain to any of the cues associated with your drug of choice. Sights, smells, brand logos, places, even mere thoughts of a favorite food can create a surge of neurotransmitter release in the reward pathways. This is amplified in the early stages of abstinence. This is why we use NMF as short for "not my food" in the online BLE community as opposed to naming specific addictive foods. In the outside world, food cues are everywhere, and as a population, we know we are extra sensitive to their effects; in the BLE community, we take care of each other by maintaining at least one safe space to gather and connect without being inundated.

The forms of cognitive impairment that go along with food addiction, alas, are many. Just as alcoholics show impaired inhibition when it comes to alcohol, food addicts show impaired inhibition when it comes to food. The prefrontal cortex, which is the executive decision maker assisting with impulse control, is blunted, leading to more impulsivity and less control. During food cravings, overall thinking is compromised. And other studies have shown deficits in memory and attention.[14] One study found that early life exposure to processed foods is associated with lifelong deficits in both learning and memory.[15]

If any of this resonates with you, you are not alone. Thanks to research like this, the zeitgeist is shifting and the reality of food addiction is going from shocking and controversial to obvious and accepted.

But we're not quite there yet. A lot of people mistakenly only equate addiction with needles and living under bridges. Yet caffeine addiction is normalized and nicotine addiction is obvious. It's my hope that food addiction becomes equally normalized and obvious because you can't treat a condition you don't think you have.

Particularly for people at 6 and above on the Susceptibility Scale, there can be a huge upside to embracing the moniker. The diagnosis of "food addiction" gives us a way to work a full program of recovery that gives us the results we want. Healing from food addiction involves a lot of sacrifice and embodying a new way of living, including new daily routines. And typically, people don't invest that heavily in something unless there's a rationale and motivation for it. Thinking of yourself as a food addict very gratefully living in recovery can help fuel and sustain that recovery. I have seen so many people's lives blossom once they embraced, without judgment or stigma, that they really were food addicts.

Finally, I want to add that processed foods are probably the most socially acceptable drug (other than, perhaps, caffeine), and oftentimes a food addict who lives in a family of drug or alcohol addicts may think of themselves as the one who has it all together. Realizing that they've been an addict all along when they thought of themselves as the "good" kid while their siblings turned to drugs or alcohol can be hard for someone who's always defined themselves in contrast to the addict in their life. But neurologically it's all the same. As is stated in the textbook *Processed Food Addiction: Foundations, Assessment, and Recovery*, "The neurological evidence for overeating as an addiction is extensive."[16]

But there is another reason food addiction is so tenacious. Most of us have a part of ourselves that really wants to eat addictive foods. Not just our brain, which has been rewired to crave them, but a part of our psyche that may have been using food for years to navigate stress, to reward, to celebrate, to comfort, to soothe. That part of us is called the Food Indulger.

THE FOOD INDULGER PART

If you have an addictive relationship with food, you are probably very familiar with the part of you that experiences cravings. It could be a light, persistent thinking about your favorite "treat," a desire to hop in the car and get something in particular, or an overpowering compulsion that leads you to shovel food into your mouth until you literally can't move without pain. If you are high on the Susceptibility Scale, these addictive tendencies are probably extreme and may have impacted you for a lot of your life. If you are lower on the Susceptibility Scale, they may be milder, and you may not even consider your relationship with food to be addictive. The bottom line is that if you deal with uncontrollable food cravings, you most likely have a protective part that we in Bright Line Eating call the Food Indulger.

Your Food Indulger is unique to you. In Parts Work, we personify our parts and build imaginative relationships with them. We learn their stories and their motivations. For many of us, they come alive and will listen to us. They can also be negotiated with.

One of the reasons that Parts Work ties in so well with BLE is that BLE is structured around abstinence from the primary addictive foods—sugar and flour. It's a way of relating to food that, when followed, will allow you to release weight, move past physical cravings, and eventually settle into your Bright Body. Because of this, it's very easy to notice parts of you that are wanting you to veer away from the structure. If your Authentic Self is running the show, BLE feels effortless. When BLE feels challenging, it's because parts of you are getting activated and trying to interfere.

When we start BLE, there is a detox period in our brain where physical cravings for sugar and flour gradually fade away. Automaticity kicks in, and it starts to become easy to not snack and to only eat three meals a day. But we also know that food cravings can have an emotional component to them. This is the Food Indulger.

The Food Indulger is the part that protected us from pain, or stress, or any other uncomfortable emotion by using food. It offered us food to soothe, to celebrate, and to numb out. The image of someone deep in a quart of ice cream after a breakup is a common sitcom trope. But many of us go into the food in order to avoid emotions or manage stress. Many of us have built eating into the way we handle nearly everything hard in our life. And we are socialized to do that. Think about the weight gain people half-jokingly called the COVID-19. There was a societal agreement that eating processed food was how we were going to cope with the pandemic.

This is also a common coping mechanism among over-achievers or over-caretakers, who depend on the extra food to fuel their stress-filled lives. Sugar- and flour-based snacks and treats, or simply grazing nonstop, are the crutches they use to get through the day.

Many successful people feel frustrated that they've been high achievers in other areas of their lives and don't understand why they haven't been successful with managing their weight. The reason is that their dysfunctional relationship with food is part of what allows them to achieve so much. It offsets the tremendous stress they are under.

So even after the physical cravings have gone away, your Indulger might be trying all sorts of strategies to get you to eat off-plan in order to deal with the stress or other uncomfortable emotions in your life. It's important to know that your Food Indulger is trying to help you, even if its strategy is ultimately unhelpful. The variety of positive intentions that our Food Indulgers might have include: filling up a feeling of emptiness inside, numbing strong feelings, providing some physical pleasure, having some fun, rewarding you for working hard, allowing you to not feel controlled, keeping you from falling apart, helping you suppress your anger or sadness, giving you a break or reprieve from the nonstop obligations of life, and many more.

Many Bright Lifers know that if they get back into the sugar and flour, their relapse is going to be *really* bad, so they only allow their Food Indulgers to indulge on BLE-compliant food. While this approach certainly is better, going down this path will likely impact your weight loss (or cause your weight to creep up if you're on Maintenance), and it might end up being a slippery slope back to your old default eating patterns. At the very least, you'll likely find it robs you of much of your peace and freedom.

If you notice your Food Indulger part is active, how do you calm it down without eating addictively? The first thing to notice is whether you've let sugar and flour back into your diet, because if you have, then the presence of the Food Indulger is at least partly the psychological manifestation of your physical addiction to these substances resurfacing. The solution is to get some support while you get the sugar and flour back out of your diet.

If you've been Bright for a stretch of time and you're still experiencing cravings, it's time to get curious. Is your Food Indulger part trying to help you avoid or cope with feelings? Start to notice what you are feeling when the Indulger's food cravings show up. Can you turn toward that feeling? Perhaps if you cried, journaled, or expressed the feeling directly, the Indulger's influence would lessen. Feeling and processing your feelings will calm down your Indulger. If you have past trauma that is often triggered, perhaps time with a therapist will allow the Indulger to relax. We will talk in Chapter 7 about the importance of support. The more support you have, both internal and external, the more likely you will be able to keep your Indulger from acting out.

When people have had initial success with BLE and then, for some seemingly mysterious reason, fall off the wagon, it is a sign that it's time to go deeper and do some Parts Work. Food Indulgers come in many forms, and we have a quiz in

Appendix B so you can determine what type (or types) of Indulger(s) you have. If you are curious about the role your Food Indulger might be playing in keeping you from the ease you want to experience with Bright Line Eating, Appendix B at the end of this book is an excellent place to start.

CHAPTER 3

FOOD ADDICTION IS THE HARDEST

I know I am sticking my neck out here. Please allow me to not just stick my neck out but also to climb out and stand on a box—as a recovering addict who used to be hopelessly, mercilessly hooked on crystal meth and crack cocaine. As a recovering food addict. As a brain and cognitive scientist. As a professor, a mentor, and a coach to thousands of people trying to break free from sugar and flour.

Food. Is. The. Hardest.

Nothing—not crack cocaine, alcohol, methamphetamine, cigarettes, or heroin—*nothing* is harder to beat than food.

And there are seven unique reasons why this is true.

1) Addictions are grouped into two categories: substance addictions and process or behavioral addictions. The substance of food partnered with the process of eating counts as both. Behavioral or process addictions include gambling, shopping, watching pornography, and Internet gaming. These are processes that are inherently rich, detailed, and cue-laden enough to be addictive because just engaging in the behavior leads the brain to deliver its own addictive hit of chemicals.

With highly refined foods, you are consuming a substance that is downregulating the brain within the behavioral context of a process that is rich, varied, and rewarding enough on its own to be addictive. It's delivering both.

2) The drive to consume food is hardwired into us to ensure that we survive. Unique among all substances, the target of our addiction in this case hijacks an already existing survival mechanism wired in at the deepest level to have the biggest import. You don't need alcohol to survive, and you weren't hardwired to make alcohol procurement and consumption part of your every waking thought, but that's exactly how we were wired to think about food.

On top of that, so many "foods" today are akin to what the psychological literature calls supranormal stimuli. Scientists have found that songbirds will abandon their natural, pale blue eggs to go sit on fake fluorescent blue eggs that are so big that the birds continually slide off.[17] This is a perfect example of a supranormal stimulus. If you think about an orange slushy compared to an actual orange found in nature, it's a garish exaggeration of what actual food is. And when these jacked-up "foods" take over our built-in survival circuitry, it's game over.

3) Food addiction has the brutal side effect of excess weight, and losing weight can trigger food addiction. Imagine, for a moment, a universe in which drinking alcohol gave you horrible, disfiguring acne. Not just disfiguring acne but *fatal* acne. You stop drinking. Then you need to address the acne, or you'll live with it for your whole life and meet a premature death. But the only treatments that get rid of the acne come with the side effect of reawakening your desire to drink again.

That is the bind many people coming into food recovery face. Food addiction usually, though not always, involves the accumulation of excess adipose tissue. And the issue with having a weight problem is that the brain evolved to protect us against weight loss. It defends against theoretical impending starvation by creating biological and hormonal changes: for example, increasing ghrelin, a hunger hormone; decreasing leptin, a satiety hormone; and decreasing thyroid hormones, which regulate the metabolism. Any of these hormonal changes can trigger relapse, and all of them together make staying on the wagon exceedingly hard.

No other addiction creates an ancillary side effect that lives on long after you've stopped using, a side effect that is, in and of itself, unhealthy to live with unaddressed. And when you try to address it, it triggers relapse to the initial primary addiction. It's a confounding loop to get stuck in.

Think about it: healing the liver doesn't cue the brain to make you want to drink. Clearing the lungs doesn't cue the brain to make you want to smoke. But steadily losing a lot of weight can cue the brain to send you on another lose-and-regain cycle that inevitably results in weighing more than you did when you started and *still* being addicted to food. It might just be the most vicious of vicious circles.

4) You can't just stop. Food isn't cigarettes. Or alcohol. Or heroin. You can't just quit. It's a substance that you have to keep consuming, which is torturous and maddening.

Imagine if you went to an AA meeting and got a sponsor, and the first thing they told you is how you'd need to choose a drink to have for breakfast, say a shot of vodka, but only 2.0 ounces, no more. Then a drink for lunch, maybe one glass of red wine, weighed and measured. And then one drink for dinner as well.

Needing to eat creates the issue of actually knowing when you're sober. What does recovery even look like? The line between an addictive food and a nonaddictive food is, A, not always clear and, B, at least somewhat unique to the individual. And this lack of certainty about where the lines are creates a slippery slope that can lead to relapse.

We get dozens of emails every day asking granular questions about what's permissible in Bright Line Eating. We've codified our basic food plan and have hundreds of answers in our FAQ data bank. But there is a huge variance in the human animal, every predilection is on a bell curve, and a food that is neutral for one person is very often a trigger for another. This is where I invite everyone to be a scientist by objectively observing their own responses and behaviors and finalizing their own program based on their personal biology. And, most certainly, belonging to a community that has very strong shared norms around what foods to abstain from will help tremendously. But make no mistake: the fact that you can't just abstain entirely makes food recovery astronomically harder.

5) The multitrillion-dollar food industry is very invested in our ongoing addiction. There are still no limits on soda commercials, sugar cereal commercials, candy commercials, or fast-food commercials aimed at kids. It can feel like every billboard, every road sign, every poster in a storefront window is depicting stretched cheese and some kind of tagline about how much you deserve it. Remember, the food addict's brain is extra sensitive to these cues.

The food industry is now using medical and neuroscience technologies like functional magnetic resonance imaging (fMRI) to track how to amplify our hedonic response to their products. Essentially, this means putting food addicts in fMRI machines and then watching their brains as they're shown various commercials and as they try various formulations of snack foods, sugary foods, and junk foods. Food companies can then alter the taste of their outrageously delicious industrial products and market them ever more effectively.[18]

Simply living in the world is a minefield for relapse, which is just not the case if, say, you're recovering from heroin addiction. Driving to work doesn't come with an endless series of invitations to shoot heroin, but it does come with an endless series of enticements to eat exactly the foods that you know you shouldn't be eating.

6) Food addiction is triggered by more temporal cues and location cues than any other addiction. Think about how often the food addict eats, compared to, say, how often the heroin addict shoots heroin. Then think about how many places you're allowed, even encouraged, to eat, compared to, say, how many places you're allowed to smoke cigarettes. Food is unparalleled in its frequency of consumption and unlimited range of places for consumption. Why does this matter?

Well, to develop an addiction, you first need an underlying susceptibility. This can be caused by genetics or a rough childhood or both. But even with that underlying susceptibility, you have to wire up addiction in a certain domain. For example, I'm as addictable as they come, but I have developed zero shopping addiction thus far in my life. I would still be eligible to develop a shopping addiction if, for example, I was going through the death of a loved one and I was aching, and I found that a trip to the mall really helped and then I went again. But I would have to wire up the experience of ache and longing and pain followed by relief and all the cues of shopping that go along with that.

Addiction gets wired into our brains through repeat experiences with the drugs that are associated with a time and place. Cigarette smoking would be the next closest to food in these terms because a three-packs-a-day smoker smokes all day long in any permissible setting. And certain actions, like finishing a meal or walking out of a movie theater, would be absolutely powerful cues to smoke a cigarette that would plague a former smoker for months and even years after quitting smoking.

But for the recovering food addict, it's so much worse. Smoking and drugs are prohibited in many places, while eating is hardly prohibited anywhere. Even a chain-smoker can't smoke in an elevator, in a movie theater, or on an airplane, but two out of three of those locations involve active invitations to eat addictive foods. Essentially, the range and scope of temporal cues and location cues for food turn the whole world and the whole flow of the day into a triggered reminder that it's time to abandon your recovery and eat.

7) There is social pressure not to consider food an addiction, and there are hardwired social drives to eat. Let's face it: a lot of the people we know are also addicted to food, and collective addiction promotes an ethos of, "Come on, you're being too extreme. Don't worry about it. You've got to eat all foods in moderation." This attitude is everywhere, and if you continue on the path of food recovery for long enough, you will absolutely experience pushback from the social environment.

I've been to many a place on New Year's Eve over my 27 years of sobriety and said some version of, "No champagne for me, thank you. I don't drink." And I've watched how the responses have changed over the years. It's now really easy to decline alcohol, and people will stumble over themselves to get me a seltzer and make me feel comfortable. Not so if I say, "No, thank you. I don't eat sugar," when the pumpkin pie is passed at Thanksgiving. People do not see that choice in the recovery paradigm, and they do not hold the same kind of respect for it.

Furthermore, bonding over food is hardwired into our social brains, our very ways of experiencing belonging and community. Alcoholics who stop drinking often ache with the loss of their drinking buddies, the bar where everyone knows their name. But once fully sober, they find plentiful associations with groups of people who are not blending consumption of liquor with their hours of harmonious association. But essentially all gatherings of people, everywhere, find ways big and small to blend consumption of food with their mutual fellowship. And learning to do it differently, to not partake of addictive eating while still feeling like you belong, is very, very hard.

I say all of this not to exhaust or demoralize you but to remind you that what we are up against is vast on every front—from the challenges in our own brain to the challenges that come at us from society at large. The shifts that have taken place in our food environment in recent years have created a set of conditions that put those of us who are highly susceptible to food addiction in quite a predicament.

To find our way forward, we are going to need a lot of support and a total reframe on the very nature of food recovery.

Most likely, the supports we've been working with thus far have been insufficient. For most of us (even though we weren't aware of it), the only thing we have had to manage our addiction, control our cravings, or keep our Food Indulger in check is a part of us called the Food Controller. The Food Controller manages our food, starts diets, and pushes us to comply with the rules. When we're on a streak of success with our food, it's also the part of us that gets super scared about it all unraveling before our eyes.

THE FOOD CONTROLLER PART

The next part you need to meet is your Food Controller. Whereas your Food Indulger wants to use food to comfort and distract you from stress and pain, your Food Controller is the part of you that wants to restrict, limit, and stick to the plan. Your Food Controller is probably the part of you that has you reading this book right now. People with strong Food Controllers tend to love Bright Line Eating because it's so clear and structured.

Do you tend to start a project in a structured way and see it through to completion? Does it bother you when things are out of order? Do you need to control situations or other people? The people who tend to be more run by their controlling parts are the list keepers and the perfectionists. On the other hand, if you are more freewheeling, rebellious, or spontaneous, then you are probably run by other parts we'll meet later. In Internal Family Systems, we seek to befriend and heal our parts, which allows us to live our life from our Authentic Self. Our Authentic Self can naturally ride that balance between control and spontaneity.

The Food Controller tends to treat us the way we were treated as kids. Did you have harsh, shaming, and strict parents? You might find that your Food Controller uses that exact same strategy in trying to control your Food Indulger. Were you raised with little supervision and with permissive parenting? You might find your Food Controller having a very permissive style full of bargaining, such as, "You can't eat that, but you can have this," or, "Okay, but just a little."

People in treatment will often say they feel like they *only* have a Food Indulger and wish they had a Food Controller to get them back on track. Their Food Controller has given up. People with weak or permissive Food Controllers need external support. It works like this: Your Food Indulger responds to stress or underlying pain, and the cravings start. Once your Food Indulger is activated, your Food Controller will try to control it. The Food Controller will either be successful or it won't. If your Food Controller isn't strong enough, you can bring in more external support and accountability or, better yet, work to address the stress or underlying pain.

In Bright Line Eating, we focus on both: bringing our life more into balance and getting lots of external support. As you learn Parts Work, a third option opens up. You learn that you can dialogue and negotiate with your parts, thus changing these lifelong patterns in real time.

Like the Food Indulger, the Food Controller is just trying to help you the best way it knows how, even though it can sometimes feel like you're getting yelled at or harshly criticized from inside your own head. The noise this part can make is quite loud and can consume a lot of your internal dialogue when it's active.

This is why we visualize our parts, so we can start to feel them as separate from us. What does your Food Controller look like? Is it an executive vice president in a crisp business suit, a judge with a gavel, or perhaps a frazzled-looking parent? The support and accountability practices we cover in Chapter 7 will help bolster your Food Controller if it is feeling overwhelmed. This will allow it to release its grip because it will know it doesn't have to support you by itself.

A strong Food Controller can get you into a Bright Body, but you won't have peace until you've brought your life into balance and gotten your Food Indulger to calm down. In Parts Work, we know that most of our obsessive thinking about food is actually an age-old battle between our Food Indulger and our Food Controller. When one gets stronger, the other tries to match its influence. This polarization is the "crazy" that many of us experience in our heads around our relationship with food. There are as many different versions of this scenario as there are people, and you will have your own version of this polarization. As you start to get to know your

parts and build relationships with them, this largely uncon-
scious process will start to become visible to you.

Once you can start to notice the interplay between these
two parts, it becomes easier to run your program from your
Authentic Self. This brings the real freedom and neutrality
around food that so many of us seek. Automaticity sets in and
we cruise through our life, free of food thoughts, living in our
Bright Body, and able to take the day as it comes.

CHAPTER 4

THE REZOOM REFRAME

After reading Baumeister and Tierney's book *Willpower* and getting that guidance to write a book called *Bright Line Eating* during my morning meditation, I named the four boundaries that form the scaffolding for my food recovery my Bright Lines. In Bright Line Eating, we make a commitment to four nonnegotiable boundaries: sugar, flour, meals, and quantities. As a vegetarian commits to not eating meat, we commit to not eating sugar or flour, in any form, ever. We commit to eating only meals—for most of us that's three per day—with not so much as a carrot stick in between. Not to be rigid but to be clear. And we commit to only eat certain quantities of food, so we never have to second-guess ourselves.

Bright Lines. Firm boundaries that, paradoxically, set us free.

You've probably used bright lines in the past, even if you've never done Bright Line Eating. Perhaps you needed a bright line for your ex-boyfriend (*no texting Johnny anymore*), or a bright line for nicotine, or maybe even a bright line for something as serious as cutting or purging, something you realize you can *never* do again.

For those of us who have brains that are more susceptible to food addiction—to cravings, to obsession about what we've eaten or not eaten, to excessive focus on how we're doing with our weight and our food—Bright Lines can produce a lot of freedom.

But here's the rub: they can also produce a lot of perfectionism.

Now, maybe you've never tried an abstinence-based approach to food recovery, but you've probably experienced perfectionism

51

in other realms. Maybe when you started to work out, you were determined never to miss a workout. Or you started to meditate, and you meditated every morning. Or perhaps you decided to follow some other kind of food system, and you obsessed about when you were on track with it and when you'd fallen off the wagon.

I want to present an entirely new way of thinking about being on a food journey that gets away from the black-and-white, all-or-nothing paradigm of either we're sticking to this perfectly or we've fallen off the wagon and are absolutely lost and demoralized. First, let me show you some pictures that help illustrate the problem with that old way of thinking. This graph represents our success with whatever food program we're following. This is what is going to happen over time. We launch our endeavor with a lot of fanfare, a lot of motivation, and a lot of excitement, like a New Year's resolution. And because we're super motivated, our success skyrockets at the very beginning.

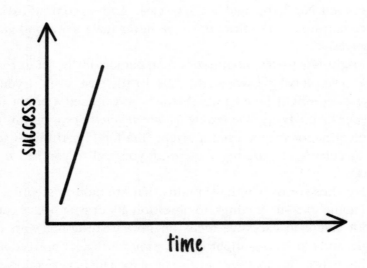

Our growing sense of accomplishment is palpable. The weight is melting off. Confidence and positive emotions are flying high.

Then it's been a couple of months. Maybe we go on a cruise, or a family member gets sick, and we start to relapse. There's this moment of awareness—or panic—that we've fallen off track. For many of us, there's a sinking feeling of horror that comes with cresting the peak and crashing back down.

Our success sharply decreases over a short period of time, and before we know it, we've plummeted down and entered the Danger and Destruction Zone. This is where we're hurting bad. Often, there's a lot of hiding, numbing out, procrastinating, and fuzzy thinking. In my experience, in this zone I can gain back all my excess weight, hardly even realizing that the weeks and months are passing.

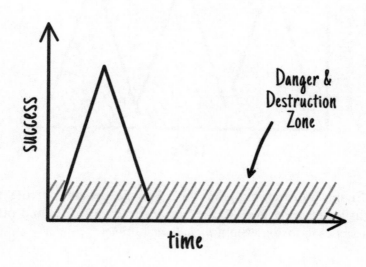

For many of us, once we reach the Danger and Destruction Zone, we're not going to restart again until we get really, really "sick and tired of being sick and tired" and somehow, some way, a new feeling of motivation is born in us. We resolve to start over, maybe with a plan or program we've done in the past but with a commitment to really make it work this time. Or maybe we scrap the old plan for a new one. But either way, now we make another new attempt, with its corresponding big launch and the accompanying need to do it perfectly.

And then the crash. Again.

On and on this goes—the really painful crash-and-burn cycle of food addiction.

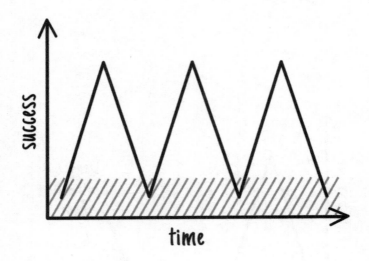

In our research program, the average person starting the Bright Line Eating Boot Camp has tried various diets and other approaches to losing weight *more than 16 times*.

We need to end this cycle. It's too destructive—to our morale and our bodies. We need a Rezoom Reframe.

THE REZOOM REFRAME

One of the moments that first helped me conceptualize the Rezoom Reframe took place in a hotel room. I think I was in Nashville. I had eaten something off my plan. As I sat there, I realized that my breaks and restarts weren't really painful anymore. Then I thought back on the eight years of "perfect" unbroken food recovery that I'd experienced a few years prior. As I thought about that time period deeply, I remembered that periodically, I'd actually go through times when I was doing a lot of things with my food that felt unclean or semi out of control, like relying on super big fruit, dumping cinnamon all over my breakfast cereal, or going to restaurants and ordering French fries and eating too many of them and counting them as my grain serving. Each time, I'd make a call to my sponsor, clean up my act, and get on the upswing again. I wasn't considering it a break in my Bright Lines, but I was undeniably slipping with my food.

What I realized in that hotel room was that, in a way, I had been relapsing. I just hadn't been naming it as such.

Then I started to think more deeply about the word *relapse*. It's made up of two pieces, the prefix "re-" and the stem "lapse," lapse being a period of time when things have gone offtrack a bit. It's not the end of the world, and, in fact, it's a very natural part of life. That's when I visualized what the ebbs and flows feel like when you're maintaining your food recovery over the years. It's not that there aren't ups and downs with your program. It's just that they feel smoother, with gentle curves between the ups and downs rather than sharp angles, and they are maintained at a higher level of success, above the Danger and Destruction Zone.

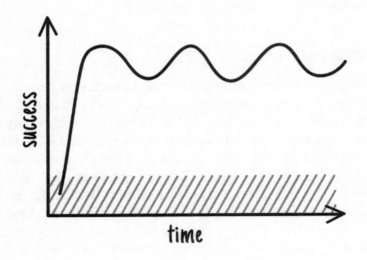

THE SHIFTS

In order to turn the crash-and-burn cycle into a much gentler sine wave, the Rezoom Reframe involves three life-changing shifts. The first is smoothing off the edges so that instead of a painful spike and crash, the cycle becomes more like rounded waves, born of a lot of acceptance and living in your Authentic Self. The second shift is learning to get back on track faster, after just a small downslide instead of a full-on crash. And the final shift involves raising the whole wave up to a higher level of success, creating a sweet and oh-so-important cushion between the bottom of each trough and the Danger and Destruction Zone. This is what's possible when you embrace the Rezoom Reframe.

After the epiphany in the hotel room, I became curious about whether long-term successful people in Bright Line Eating had also experienced lapse phases and gotten back on track. I reached out to my research team, and I asked them, "In our follow-up research program, of the people who are living in a Bright Body with Bright

Line Eating, what percent of them have broken their Bright Lines and had to rezoom?"

They ran the analysis and said, "In the Boot Camp, we ask people this set of questions every week. 'In this past week, on a scale from 1 to 7, how well did you stick with each of the following four Bright Lines: Sugar, Flour, Meals, and Quantities?' Of the thousands of people who've given us their data, not one of them has ever given themselves a score of 7 out of 7 for all four Bright Lines through the entire Boot Camp."

So the answer is 100 percent. One hundred percent of people that we have data for in Bright Line Eating have had at least a tiny lapse and had to rezoom at some point.

When these data came in and I shared them with my community, one of my Bright Lifers got really upset. She reached out to me and said, "Susan, you're wrong. I was one hundred percent perfect during the Boot Camp!" And I said, "Did you fill out all the surveys?" She said she had. So I said, "Well, we have your data, and at some point, you scored yourself at least a 6 out of 7 on something. Maybe you went to a potluck. Maybe you went to a restaurant. Maybe you went to a party, and at the end of the night, you thought, *You know what? I don't know that my quantities were perfect. Say 6 out of 7 this week for the quantities Line.* You counted it as a Bright Line Day, but that week, you gave yourself 6 out of 7 for quantities, perhaps." And she said, "Oh, yeah. I could have done that."

CRYSTAL VASES AND TEDDY BEARS

In one of the later modules of the Bright Line Eating Boot Camp, I talked about how some people might have reached a point where the Bright Line Eating journey feels really effortless. Downright *easy*. Essentially, I said, "If that's happening for you, if Bright Line Eating feels easy, here's what I want you to know: One day at a time, through weeks and weeks of not eating sugar, not eating flour, and putting your food on the scale, you've created a prized Waterford Crystal Vase. It's very valuable. *Don't juggle it.* It can break, and when it breaks, it never goes back together quite the same way. Stay grateful. Keep doing what you're doing." Which is why some people in Bright Line Eating call themselves Crystal Vasers.

Now, I want to clear something up right here: the Crystal Vase is their *recovery*, not them as a person. And the reason it's precious and worth protecting has to do with our brain.

When our food has been in order for a long stretch of weeks, months, or years, an interesting phenomenon emerges where the brain starts to shield us from deviating from our food plan by actively inhibiting any impulse to do so, in the way two magnets will actively repel each other if you try to put the positive or negative ends together. It's almost as if, by deeply accepting the identity of a Bright Lifer, our brain comes to believe that it's imperative for our life and our well-being that we not deviate from our food plan.

When we back that up with a long string of successful actions, it starts to seem as if we can't take that bite of sugar or flour, even if we vaguely wanted to. And I use that word "vaguely" on purpose, because at this point, true cravings are a thing of the past. Now we just have these gossamer thoughts that we can easily brush away. If we ever seriously considered eating something off our food plan, we'd find it would be really hard to actually eat it now.

But this is what I and thousands of other people in our community have experienced: the moment we take a bite off our food plan, the moment we deliberately, willfully cross that line and decide, *You know what? Screw it. I'm gonna eat whatever I want tonight*, it's the equivalent of shattering the vase.

What happens then is the magnets reverse, and they pull together with a force that feels impossible to stop. Whether immediately or after a few days, or perhaps a month or two (if we're lower on the Susceptibility Scale), the food that once used to be so safely out of bounds now calls so loudly, and the behavioral impulse to eat it is so intense and overwhelming that we find ourselves simply unable to resist.

In my investigations of the way the brain works, I've come to believe that this must be governed by the basal ganglia. In his book, *The Hungry Brain*, Dr. Stephan Guyenet explains that when it comes to selecting the next action for us to execute, the basal ganglia act as if they're bouncers in front of an exclusive nightclub, keeping out some patrons and admitting others. At any given moment there are hundreds of things we could do next—a nearly infinite array of options that could be paralyzing. So the basal ganglia scan the crowd and only let in the top options.

After we have adhered to our food plan for a nice long stretch of time, we enter a merciful state where the bouncer portion of the basal ganglia doesn't even allow eating off-plan to enter the realm of possibility. Any actions involving eating when it's not mealtime or eating foods that are most definitely not on the plan simply aren't allowed in past the exclusive red velvet rope. They are actively kept out of consideration. The specific neural pathway in the basal ganglia that likely regulates this state is aptly named the NoGo pathway.

But once we eat one of those outrageously rewarding processed poison treats, the resulting flood of dopamine activates the "Go" pathway, which suppresses the "NoGo" pathway, and bam— we're back in the land where our willpower is woefully insufficient to fend off the beast. The food thoughts are now jumping and screaming in the bouncer's face. And because the nucleus accumbens, the seat of addiction, is literally a part of the basal ganglia, they now get *preferentially* let into the club. Every time.

When we find ourselves in a brain state where sticking to our food plan has become really easy, it behooves us to remember how precious that is and how easy it is to lose it.

After I was struggling with my Bright Lines for a while, wondering if I even had the chops to lead the Bright Line Eating movement, I shot a video where I said, "I don't have a Crystal Vase anymore. I shattered it. My food recovery is more like my teddy bear, Wraucetur, who's been with me since I was six. He has no eyes because my daughter plucked them out when she was two. And he has no face because our dog chewed it off when she was a puppy. But Wraucetur is amazing, and beautiful, and cuddly. He's valuable because of our history, and because I never forsake him."

Now, as a psychologist I know that in retrospect, if you've counted something as a Bright Line Day, it gets whitewashed in your memory with the paintbrush of perfection, like all the other Bright Line Days. But the reality is that even someone who's built this glorious, shiny, sparkly vase of Bright Line Eating diligence has been on some kind of cycle of very slight lapsing and rezooming all along. The difference between having Crystal Vase Recovery and Teddy Bear Recovery is that if you have a Crystal Vase, the downslope never crashes into the Danger and Destruction Zone. And the edges are a little bit smoothed off. The ride is gentler. There's cushion.

I want everyone to have that cushion.

THE SCIENCE BEHIND THE REFRAME

In the old paradigm, when we broke our Lines, we instantly feared weight regain. We feared that everything we'd worked so hard to achieve was about to unravel in front of our eyes. We questioned the new identity we'd built up, meal by meal, day by successful day, and feared that we might not be that successful person we were starting to hope that we could be. That's a pretty scary turning point, a situation worthy of fear and panic.

Now let's look at how fear and panic work in the brain. There's a network of areas that are involved in a fear response, and first we're going to focus on the amygdala, a tiny almond-shaped part that sits deep inside the brain. It's a pretty primitive, primal cluster of nuclei that evolved to ensure our survival by constantly seeking out threats and priming us to fight or flee them.

When the amygdala has determined that we are in danger, the body floods with a sympathetic nervous system reaction. Our attention narrows, our bronchial tubes dilate, and our hearts start to pound so we can pump fresh oxygen to our muscles to run as fast as possible.

But here's the thing: Once the amygdala perceives a threat, it sends a signal up to our executive control center, the cortex, for evaluation, to ask, "Am I really in danger?" The dorsal anterior cingulate cortex will amplify the fear signal if, in fact, you're actually in danger. And the ventromedial prefrontal cortex will dampen that fear signal if you're not really in danger.

To see how this works, imagine you're in a haunted house and something hairy and bloody jumps out at you. Your brain and body will launch a fear response for a second, but then the part of your brain that knows you're in a haunted house is going to take over and remind the amygdala that you're not really in danger, and you're going to laugh and say, "Oh, that one was intense. It got me." You might experience the initial flood of hormones, but the full cascade would be pulled back in.

This is why, from a conceptual standpoint, the framework that we're operating under matters so much. Do we believe that we are now on a downward slope that's irreversible and we're going to crash and burn and gain back all our weight? Or do we operate from the Rezoom Reframe, where a downward slope is inevitable, safe, and predictable because we're human beings and we live in a world where we know how to catch it before we crash into the Danger and Destruction Zone?

Understanding this natural pattern actually gives us the power to get off the painful, dangerous version of the roller coaster, and onto a smooth, easygoing merry-go-round, where we're always going up and down but the journey feels more controlled.

And control is key.

Research has been done with people who experience anxiety in a particular situation where other people don't. For example, air travel. Some people like flying on airplanes, while others absolutely hate it. The difference is one of perceived control. People who love flying report that they feel completely in control. They say, "I've got my laptop. I've got my movies. I love being in an airplane. I'm completely in control." Whereas the people who hate flying report feeling entirely out of control. For that whole flight, they're thinking, "We could drop out of the sky at any moment, and there's nothing I could do about it. The moment I stepped on this plane, I abdicated all control."

In our old model, the cycle of relapsing and then starting a new plan is characterized by a perception of being out of control. Once you're on the downward slope, you have no control over how fast it's going to unravel, how deep and painful the slide is going to be, and how much weight you're going to regain.

Instead, the Rezoom Reframe gives you back control because you'll learn how to smooth off the edges, how to get out of "lapse" mode and back into "rezoom" mode before you've lost too much ground, and how to raise the slope so you can turn this painful, jagged experience into a predictable way of traveling.

TWO-PRONGED APPROACH

Mastering that way of traveling involves learning two paradigms—one internal, one external. The internal paradigm is the Parts Work that Everett is teaching you at the end of each chapter. This gives you the skills to map your internal landscape as you come up against resistance or self-sabotage. The external paradigm is the Rezoom System, which is made up of three components: food, actions, and support. We will cover these in turn over the next three chapters.

THE FINAL SHIFTS

One final note before we move on.

Once the Rezoom Reframe is internalized—meaning you've learned the Rezoom System, have begun noticing how your parts come into play, and the dips down into the Danger and Destruction Zone have stopped—you'll likely notice a couple of gradual shifts taking place.

In our Bright Line Eating community, for those deeply embracing this reframe on food addiction and food recovery, here's what we've found. First, the amplitude of the sine wave decreases so that the ups and downs become even more gentle. We no longer feel like we're living in the Himalayas with high highs and low lows. It's not only smoothed out, but we feel ever more agency and control.

Best of all, as the food and weight problems melt away, we have even more capacity to grow and develop in other areas of our life. And those investments start to yield dividends. We flourish and our life satisfaction climbs. We invest in our relationships, our hobbies, our self-care, and our careers. Our focus turns to supporting and loving the people around us. In essence, we're on a slightly undulating upward trajectory.

And it never stops getting better. Not that there aren't hard times, difficult lessons, and bad days. But overall, as we adapt and grow, we feel up to the challenge: fully transformed, and finally, mercifully, *Bright*.

That is why the arrow continues upward on the cover of this book.

When I first introduced the Rezoom Reframe to the Bright Line Eating community, many people loved the model right away and saw a huge value in it. But there were also people, primarily our Crystal Vasers, who really didn't like it. They interpreted the "lapses" as giving them license to break their Lines or get loose in their program, or worse.

Let me be really clear. The Rezoom Reframe is *not* permission to break your Bright Lines. It's *not* an invitation to eat addictively. As a matter of fact, the higher you are on the Susceptibility Scale, the more important it will be to your overall peace and success that you raise your sine wave high enough that your lapses don't dip down into the Danger and Destruction Zone—the zone where you're breaking your Lines. However, the model still holds. It is an acknowledgment that lapses, in some form, happen to all of us sometimes, and the point is to stay aware and catch them early.

But take a moment to notice something. If you had that line of thinking at any point—that the reframe was giving you permission to eat a little of this or a little of that because you can just rezoom and get back on track—that wasn't your Authentic Self having that thought. It was your Food Indulger. And if you had a thought or a voice that came in right after that saying it's just not wise to embrace any framework that minimizes eating off-plan, that was your Food Controller.

Learning about your parts, which you have begun to do at the end of the last two chapters, will help you begin to unhook both the Food Indulger and the Food Controller from your food choices. In order to deepen that work, it will be incredibly important to take care of yourself—something many people in food recovery have a hard time prioritizing. This is because we often put everyone else's needs ahead of our own, and the only way we know how to take care of ourselves is by letting our Indulger soothe us.

Understanding our Caretaker and allowing it to shift some of that wonderful energy and focus onto ourselves can be a big first step in allowing our Indulger to step back.

THE CARETAKER PART

How focused is your life on other people's needs? Are you unable to say no when asked to do something for someone else? Is there little to no time for your own self-care? Do others' needs just seem more important than yours? If this sounds familiar, you are probably being run by the Caretaker.

The Bright Line Eating community is full of people with strong caretaking parts. People with strong caretaking parts usually have an overactive Food Indulger that has historically helped them fuel the caretaking work they are doing with sugar, snacks, and grazing. Their Indulger tells them they deserve a treat, that they are doing so much for everyone else, or that they really need this food to get through the day.

The Caretaker might also have you break your Lines because it doesn't want you to hurt someone's feelings by rejecting their homemade treat. Or it might keep you from leaning on family support because it doesn't want you to burden them. Or it might encourage you to eat off-plan at a dinner party rather than risk offending the host.

If we are able to be honest about our caretaking parts, we will see that most of their impulses are unhealthy codependence, creating other parts that hold a lot of resentment about the unreciprocated amount of work we do for others. It's a miserable state of affairs. If you've built up an identity as the rescuer or the hero, it can be hard to consider letting it go. But the power of Parts Work can really help. As you get to know your caretaking part, you can start to invite your Authentic Self to run your day instead.

Sometimes we are in a phase of life where there is a lot of overwhelm. It is so important to know that it is possible to be successful in Bright Line Eating during these times. If you have a strong Caretaker part that is driving you into exhaustion and overwhelm, it is critical to start doing less for others and start taking care of yourself. Stop doing unhealthy caretaking, whether it's stepping in to help someone who could help themselves or insinuating yourself into a situation to feel calm and in control but making a lot of work for yourself in the process.

Reflect for a moment: How much unhealthy caretaking are you doing? How much time would you have for yourself if you stopped it? Next, gradually let go of all the things you are doing out of guilt or obligation. You can also eliminate the word *yes* from your vocabulary. Replace it with *no, maybe,* or *I'll get back to you about that.* If you stopped saying yes automatically, how many invitations and obligations would you decline? Give yourself permission to pause before answering.

Your time in life is precious, so spend it on things that light you up and bring you joy.

In Appendix B you will find **descriptions of the various Caretaker archetypes, plus quizzes and worksheets** to help you explore your Caretaker and the role it may have played in your life. These activities can help you shift the amount of time you spend in unhealthy caring for others, particularly caring they could do for themselves to their own benefit. Furthermore, stepping out of those roles will free up needed time and energy to focus on your own recovery as we learn the Rezoom System, which is what we're going to cover next.

CHAPTER 5

FOOD

Now that you understand why food addiction is so tenacious, we're going to shift our attention to the three categories of choices and behaviors that make up the Rezoom System: food, actions, and support.

Food is the foundational layer, the first thing we have to bring our attention back to when we're rezooming. To kick off the topic of food, I want to first address the fact that your food might not be Bright right at this very moment. If you've never done Bright Line Eating before and are curious to see if it could do for you what it has done for thousands of others, you'll need the basics of the program, which you can find in the book *Bright Line Eating* or at BrightLineEating.com, where we can guide you through getting started step-by-step online. But if you've been in some form of food recovery before, the starting place for rezooming is a reexamination of your food habits and practices.

This means I'm going to be inviting you at each turn to reengage with the foundational habits and practices—things like doing regular food prep or writing down your food the night before. Have you been doing them? If not, how come? If only partially, why? Could there be a part of you that is interfering with your commitment to living Bright?

I'm going to be coming at this material with all the insight that I've gained in the six years since I created the Boot Camp. I constantly receive feedback on coaching calls and in response forms, YouTube comments, emails, and Facebook posts, and I pay attention and keep adjusting how I teach these concepts. Whether you are new to Bright Lines or have already embraced Bright Line Eating in your life, it is important to dive into these concepts anew as an integral component of the Rezoom Reframe.

NOT ALL BRIGHT DAYS ARE CREATED EQUAL

Language is all categorization, meaning that in our brains, words denote categories. One of the jobs of the language learner is to figure out, "What's the category of things this word refers to?" At Bright Line Eating, we've defined the category of a successful day, food-wise, as a Bright Line Day.

We know from the psychology of categorization that when items are put into the same category, the mind blurs them to be more similar to each other. And when items are put into separate categories, the mind shifts them to be more different from each other.

What this means is that in your Bright Line Eating journey, you have stopped really noticing the differences among your Bright Line Days because your brain categorizes them as all the same. You head into bed thinking, *That was a Bright Line Day. Chalk it up. Adding another day to the tally.* But Bright Line Days are not all created equal.

Let me spin you a scenario.

I could make a Bright Line breakfast by weighing out my portion of dry oats, adding water and a dash of salt and microwaving it, putting my precisely weighed amount of yogurt and blueberries on top, adding my exact portion of ground flaxseeds, and then bringing it to the table and eating it.

Or I could say, "You know what? I'm having a day. It's only seven-thirty A.M., but I can already tell—I need some breakfast sausage." And I could cook up a bunch of pork sausages and decide to eat them with some leftover hash browns that David made for the kids. Yes, I know he cooked those with a stick of butter. But I'm pretending I don't even notice that. I'm still weighing my exact portion of sausage and hash browns—because I'm not breaking my Bright Lines, mind you. And now I need to pick some fruit, but blueberries won't do the trick. I'm hunting around for the biggest banana I can find. You know what? This banana is still too small, so I'm going to grab another one and I'm going to weigh 6 ounces of banana, just to make sure I get every morsel of banana I'm entitled to. So now I'm having a banana and a half, because that's what it took to get 6 ounces, I've got my greasy sausage and hash browns, and I'm sitting down to eat my breakfast.

That's a Bright Line breakfast. But it's not the same as the first Bright Line breakfast. You see the distinction?

Before going to a restaurant, I could look at the menu online, talk to my sponsor or Accountability Buddy, run through the options, pick the simplest choice, ask the waiter to bring the salad undressed, and top it at the table with oil and vinegar, using my teaspoon to measure the oil carefully. Or I could just order a salad, make sure there are no croutons on it—because that's the Bright Line—but let them put the dressing on it. And now we're doing a one-plate rule for dinner. How much cheese can I put on one plate? Seriously. You get my drift.

In the sine wave of food, we all have our ways of letting things get a little slippery. Maybe it's not even a lapse in willingness, and maybe your food stays immaculate. Maybe you simply get pressed for time or resources and suddenly your Sunday, which you normally use for weekly food prep, got hijacked by life and you feel like you're on the downslope, not of your own accord.

Whatever the reason, I've been on this journey for long enough and I've coached for long enough to know that not all Bright Line Days are created equal. We're calling them all Bright Line Days, and that's fine. But we're missing data if we're not looking at them more closely.

INVENTORY

In thinking about your past, what has the texture, variation, and variance in your Bright Line Days been? Where have you played the angles, created wiggle room, or veered a little bit more to the edge of that category boundary? In your mind, go through the food itself—the heavy choices, the light choices. Go back through your behavior in restaurants and on special occasions. Do you advocate for yourself socially? Or do you have a hard time speaking up? Are there times where you go with something that's not as close to what you feel like you should be eating because maybe you've been socialized not to be needy or "difficult"? Do you, deep down somewhere, feel like it's selfish for you to speak up for yourself and take care of your food needs?

These are just some areas that come up for people in our community as they begin their rezoom work. I invite you to examine your actual daily choices further in Appendix A with the inventories you'll find there. I cannot recommend this step highly enough. When it comes down to it, we can't change our trajectory until we're honest about where we're starting.

TRACK IT REGULARLY

Now I want to invite you to track how Bright your days are regularly. If you use a nightly checklist, you might consider adding an item: If my day was Bright, how Bright was it on a scale from 1 to 5? Was I playing the angles and running close to the edge, or was I solidly simple, clean, and neutral? This is not for self-flagellation or self-recrimination. No, no, no. Put the stick away. This is for *information*. This is simply a feedback mechanism so we can look at the ebbs and flows of our behavior with food.

Our goal is always to get neutral—it's not bad or good. It makes me cringe when people are dieting and they talk about whether they were "bad" or "good" with their food. In French, the words for dieting are "faire attention," which means that when a French person wants to lose weight, they are literally saying, "I am paying attention." I love that because it simply behooves us to stay open to the information on the instrument panel so we can fly the plane well. It doesn't serve us to fly the plane with a blindfold on, right?

IF YOU'RE BREAKING YOUR LINES

This especially holds true if your sine wave is low enough to be regularly dipping into that Danger and Destruction Zone. We can shine the light on that too. In Appendix A, a second inventory asks you to consider when you tend to break your Lines. On what foods? Are there any foods that you might want to let go of? Nuts, nut butters, and melted cheese are the three I see the most often. In fact, when we were writing *The Official Bright Line Eating Cookbook*, the inclusion of those ingredients was quite a source of contention, and we had to add a big nut butter disclaimer. For some Bright Lifers, nut butters aren't triggering, and they are a key component in the grab-and-go breakfast recipes that are a lifesaver for our busy moms. For others, nut butters can lead to broken Lines and horrible downward spirals. I definitely invite you to shine a light on that for your own particular level of susceptibility.

As you consider the prompts in Appendix A, perhaps consider going all the way back. Can you think about what precedes even the first signs of wonkiness in your food? Are there attitudinal shifts that happen, things that occur internally that signal that you're on the way down the slope? Perhaps there are triggering people, or triggering circumstances, or triggering events, or triggering types of days at work or home that lead your attitude to shift in a way that leads to danger. Or perhaps a Rebel part of you becomes more active (we'll be meeting the Rebel part at the end of this chapter) and you start thinking negatively about food recovery in general, wishing you didn't have to do this at all. We've all had those thoughts. Recognizing any patterns can provide really useful information.

MEASURING AND MONITORING

Spot-check inventories, including the ones we've provided in Appendix A, are great tools to get a snapshot of where your program currently is and what your behavior with food has been in the past. But as the days unfold, ongoing measuring, monitoring, and tracking of your program will help you stay clear about what you're actually doing, so you avoid duping yourself or living in a blind spot. The more we can create habits and take actions that put our behavior right in front of our face, the more likely we are to course correct when needed. If you think about this in the context of the Rezoom Reframe, in order to live free within the gentle ups and downs of life, we've got to get back on track faster. We can't afford to slide all the way down into the Danger and Destruction Zone without even realizing we've been on an extended slide. As we lapse, we need to notice it and do what it takes to pull back up into rezoom mode.

This is why tracking, measuring, and monitoring your journey is a high-value activity. I do know that some people have resistance to it and feel that it's just not helpful or necessary for them. If that's been you and you could use a deeper rationale, I'm happy to oblige. I'll start by reminding you how rare it is, out in the big bad world, for people who've struggled with their weight to succeed long term. You need to think of yourself as an Olympic athlete in training; you're trying to do the un-doable. Do you think Olympic athletes start working out without having a clear training plan with defined success metrics that they measure themselves against every day? Do you think winning a medal just sort of happens? We're talking about rare air. Sustained weight loss is hard. The brain fights it. So if you want the gold medal of living free from food cravings in a healthy Bright Body, you'll need metrics and you'll need to take them seriously.

If you have historically had some resistance to regular tracking or a Nightly Checklist Sheet or a calendar where you put X's, I invite you to consider a few questions. Have you gotten the results you've wanted in the past with the way you worked your BLE program? Has it lasted? Is there a way you could modify your approach to tracking that would make it a better fit for you?

As the saying goes, if nothing changes, nothing changes. High-performance results don't just happen. They are the consequence of consistent intentionality over a long stretch of time, and that requires feedback loops. We need this information. It serves us.

It's the car that beeps to let us know we're veering out of our lane. Even though we should be looking right there and seeing it, sometimes we're not, and that tracking mechanism prevents a crash.

TWO APPROACHES TO THE FOOD

As you inventory your food using the tools in Appendix A, it might help to keep in mind that there are basically two approaches to food in Bright Line Eating. One way is tried and true. It's to JFTFP—just follow the friggin' plan. (Or perhaps the fabulous plan, the fantastic plan, or the original, the fuckin' plan, as you prefer.) This way is relatively safe because it is battle-tested. Lots and lots of people have done it, and there's a very strong correlation between how precisely someone follows this plan and how successful they are.

The other approach is to modify or change the plan in a way that feels like it works better for you. Obviously, that is a riskier thing to do because modifications are less tried and true. There's less evidence that they work. We do have people in our community who have chosen to make the modification of not writing down their food, or significantly changing the categories and quantities of their food plan, or breaking up meals or collapsing meals, or even adding alcohol into their program at weekly intervals. If you're thinking about modifying your plan in some significant way, the first thing I want you to consider is where you are on the Food Addiction Susceptibility Scale. The higher you are on the Scale, the riskier it is, in general, to make changes or modifications to the plan.

That doesn't mean it's the wrong thing to do. It just means it's riskier. And because you're rezooming, I'm assuming you have some history with breaking your Lines in a way that was creating an issue for you—more of a crash and burn than a gentle wave. So you could ask yourself, looking back at your own data, your own evidence, your own trajectory: How has it worked for you? Have you been getting the results you wanted? If you keep running a risky experiment that has not worked in the past, I invite you to get curious about that. Why do you think you keep doing that?

Is it possible that there's some sort of safety in keeping yourself in a loop of worrying about your food, thinking about your food? Is there something else in your life these food thoughts are distracting you from? If your food got clear and clean, what else in your life would you have to think about that might be harder? At least the food is a familiar problem, right? Just a thought.

If you still want to change your plan, and you're not sure whether or not it's the right thing to do, next I will walk you through a set of steps to help you discern whether this urge, this impulse to modify the Bright Line Eating plan, is your Authentic Self or your Food Indulger.

TUNING IN TO YOUR AUTHENTIC SELF

The road to freedom isn't the same for any two people. I know this on a spiritual level—and I know this as a scientist. My brain and your brain are going to need different things. When I first started offering Bright Line Eating to the world, I was blown away by the fact that some people could watch a 30-minute informational video, learn that flour and sugar are addictive, and go off to cut them out of their lives and lose their excess weight without needing the *ton* of long-term support to sustain that commitment that most people need.

Which is all to say that, even within a high-stakes recovery journey from a legitimate addiction, there are going to be differences, exceptions, and things you may feel called to do differently than I recommend or than anyone else has recommended—and they will work for you. Because you know yourself.

But (and this is a *huge* but) our Food Indulger can sometimes sound like the voice of inner wisdom. With addiction in play, there is a downside to having leeway, to crafting your own program, and that is getting stuck in a loop in your own mind, trying to think your way out of the trap of addiction and figure out your own plan of recovery, tailor-made for you.

In my experience, that can be fraught with booby traps. Because a lot of people have a Food Indulger part that masquerades as Authentic Self. It balks at certain parts of the program in the name of being ever more congruent with one's innermost self, but really its underlying motive is just wanting to eat addictive foods.

If you're food-addicted, the mind can be quite a trap. An old sponsor of mine used to look at me and say, "This isn't Figure-It-Out Anonymous." The worst thing our brains can do is talk us out of following our program, or out of our 12-Step rooms of recovery, or out of our support.

In my first couple of months of sobriety, I had been attending meetings two and three times a day. One day, I was walking to a taqueria with a guy after a meeting. We were sharing about our lives and getting to know each other, and at some point he looked at me and said, "You're pretty smart, aren't you?" At the time I was a high school dropout recently enrolled in community college, so inside I was beaming at this compliment.

I said, "I've been told that from time to time."

And he replied, "Yeah, I don't think you'll make it in recovery. I see it all the time. People who are smart, like you, they think their way right out of the rooms." In the moment, it felt like a slap, but his warning served me well.

With all that said, sometimes we really do need to modify the plan in order to make it work for us. So what I want to offer you next is an empowering, grounding perspective on making choices and discerning among options of all sorts. This set of steps will help you to discover whether it's your Authentic Self that you're hearing or just another part of yourself—a part that's maybe addicted, younger, afraid, wounded, or controlling.

As you try to discern which choice is in alignment with your truest aims for yourself, the first thing I want you to be aware of is that any one method of decision-making can be faulty. There are many ways of knowing or getting guidance: our mind, our heart, our gut, journaling, prayer, meditation, input from friends or family, trusted texts or scriptures, and norms or prevailing wisdom in society. And as a general rule: *always triangulate*.

Whether it's your heart, your gut, your mind, a book, or a friend, take the advice or guidance under advisement, and then triangulate it. Run it by the others. If something feels like it came from God, great, run it by some recovery friends. If something came from your spouse, run it through a few other filters. What does your heart say about this? What does your gut say about this? What does your mind say about this? What do your several close friends who are trustworthy say about this? What does prevailing wisdom say about this?

I want to remind you of what your Authentic Self feels like when it's in play. It's all the Cs. Your highest self feels calm. It feels confident. It feels clear. It feels curious, and it feels compassionate—toward yourself and others. It doesn't feel anxious or fearful or worried. It doesn't feel needy, clingy, clutching, exacting, or demanding.

As you're thinking about choices on your Bright journey, notice when you relax and feel calm, confident, and curious about how it's going to work out. In those moments, you're operating from your Authentic Self.

Now you have a choice to make. If you've triangulated but you're still feeling swirly and stirred up and anxious, then I want you to write out the two choices. Define them clearly. "I could do this, or I could do that." Put pen to paper, and in a sentence or so, succinctly define the two options.

Most likely there will be pros and cons on both sides. Because the reality is that life is full of choices that are equivalent trade-offs, and the pros and cons on both sides are long and significant. For example, do you keep living in New York City, where all your friends and your creative influences are, or do you move out to the countryside where you feel called because you want space and fresh air, and you want to garden? These are really different lives, and the pros and cons are significant on both sides.

So, it's not about pros and cons, and if you're still feeling swirly and unsettled, then here's the question to ask: "What kind of person do I want to be? The kind of person who makes *this* choice or the kind of person who makes *that* choice?"

Who we are is made up of the choices we have made. With our choices, we define more and more the person we will be tomorrow, the person we are becoming. So what kind of person do you want to be? The kind of person who makes this choice with these risks and rewards, with this value core? Or the kind of person who makes that choice?

If the choice at hand has to do with your food, whether to just follow the friggin' plan or embark on some deviation, I have two last things to say. The first is that trying any kind of deviation on top of an unstable foundation is not wise. If your Lines are wobbly or wonky, or you're in the first few days, 30 days, 60 days, 90 days of starting BLE or of a rezoom, that's not the time to go experimenting. You can't get clean data when you're in early recovery because your brain is not humming along at a baseline of peace that's stable enough to know if it worked or not. Whether you are beginning BLE or embarking on a major rezoom, I strongly encourage you to follow the plan as closely and precisely as possible, at the beginning, to let your brain heal.

The second thing I want to say is that the higher you are on the Susceptibility Scale and the more intense your history with food addiction is, the higher the stakes become. If you're a 5 on the Susceptibility Scale, then starting off by following the plan and later incorporating deviations will likely be a rewarding and productive way to modify Bright Line Eating for the long term. If you're a 9 or 10 on the Scale, the downside risk of even controlled experimentation is tremendous.

Nowhere is this truer than with alcohol. Alcohol is not included in the Bright Line Eating food plan because alcohol is a sugar molecule with an ethanol addition that lowers your inhibitions and makes you more susceptible to doing things that you wouldn't if you were sober. Including eating excess food.

Yet, of all the experiments I see people run, alcohol is one of the most prevalent. People want to add a glass of wine into their routine once a week or have champagne on special occasions. Whether or not it works seems to have everything to do with their Susceptibility Score. As a general rule, the cutoff I've seen is

6 and below. They are able to add in alcohol occasionally without tipping the applecart, meaning they're able to continue living in their Bright Body while remaining peaceful with food. They're not on a roller coaster of breaking and rezooming, and they're not thinking excessively about that glass of wine that they're going to have on Friday night. For people who are 7 and above, adding any alcohol to their food plan tends to become an obsessive albatross. It leads to breaks in their Lines and eventually robs them of their freedom altogether. But sometimes not right away. I've seen 7s on the Scale spend literally years running and rerunning the alcohol experiment, letting it consume an enormous chunk of their life's focus.

If your case of food addiction is that severe and you've found peace through Bright Line Eating, the first question you might want to ask yourself is whether you want to even mess with it at all. Remember—insanity is doing the same thing over and over and expecting a different result. And it's also finding what really works and then deciding to stop doing it.

THE 4 QUESTIONS REVISITED

If you've decided to deviate from the BLE food plan in some way, or perhaps you made that decision a while back and for some time now have been incorporating foods or behaviors that are not the BLE standard, you're going to need some way to determine whether it's really working for you. How can you know?

The 4 Questions will help. The 4 Questions are an inquiry process I introduced in the Bright Line Eating Boot Camp and book as a way to experiment, mindfully, with trying something that's either a minor or a major deviation from the Bright Lines and then determining whether your experiment has worked. For example, you might want to experiment with Ezekiel bread, a form of bread that technically doesn't have flour in the ingredients list. Many people have found it to be triggering, but many others eat it and it works for them. Or fill in your own example of a food that might be borderline or off the plan.

First, we ask ourselves: "Do I have peace around it? Am I obsessing about when I'm going to have it again?" When I'm eating neutral foods, I never think about my food between meals. When a food is lighting me up, I often start fantasizing about it long in advance of mealtime. That's not peace.

The second question is: "Is it healthy? Nutritionally speaking, is it adding value to my food plan?" For example, green tea matcha has some caffeine and also has one of the strongest antioxidant profiles of any food anywhere. If you're consuming the food or beverage for health reasons, that would factor in here. Similarly, if it's unhealthy or nutritionally vacuous (think rice cakes), that would be a ding here.

Third: "Is it messing with my weight? Is my weight loss proceeding on track? Or am I stable at Maintenance and right in my range where I want to be?"

And fourth: "Is it escalating?" You might try Ezekiel bread once, think you're only going to have it on the weekends, and now suddenly you're needing it every day. Or you might have one glass of red wine, and then suddenly you need another one. And now you can't attend any event without your brain whispering that you want some alcohol. One cup of coffee becomes two, becomes three.

All of which leads to an unspoken additional question that forms the foundation of the 4 Questions process. Ask yourself: "Overall, is my program working?" Because if you have that glass of wine and you don't have a second one, and you don't obsess about it all week, that seems like a successful deviation. But if, in between, you break your Lines once or twice on other things, or in general your program is not solid, you actually don't have a basis from which to say the experiment is working. *It's only working if your whole program is working.*

LIFE BEYOND FOOD

What role is food playing in your life? When Bright Line Eating is humming along at its best, food is a lovely part of the day and really no more. It's nice, like taking a hot shower is nice, but you wouldn't catch me spending the whole day in there. Food is an enjoyable, pleasurable form of fuel. But neutral.

Is that what food is for you? Or is it more? Is it the highlight of your day? Your primary form of comfort and entertainment? Of connection? Is it a way that you distract or numb yourself? If you're worried or anxious or resentful, do you get so stressed and bottled up that you're driven to the food to cope with it all?

For sure, I still use food for celebration. I think some amount of that is fine, but if I ever were to feel like I can't have a good time without "special" foods, even if they're Bright Line friendly, it would definitely be time to look at that. The question to ask is: In what other ways can I get my needs met? We need to celebrate, to connect, to comfort ourselves, to cope when we're angry, anxious, or worried. We need all of these things. But food isn't the best way to meet any of those needs. There are better, more fulfilling, more helpful ways.

STARVATION BRAIN

Neutrality around food is always the goal because it's a very peaceful way to live. When I'm in that zone, I am freed up to accomplish so much in my life. But what if food is occupying your thinking 24/7, 365? What if your three meals are absolutely the most important thing that happens in your day, by far? What if you have a brain that's constantly asking, *Is it mealtime yet? How about now?*

I call that Starvation Brain. I know what it feels like because I lived with it for a long, long time. I felt obsessed and crazy and like I was living in a little box. My days were an extended stretch of hanging out for the next meal. If you're living in that box but your Lines are Bright and the weight's coming off, I want to let you know it *will* pass. You will get down to Maintenance, you will get food added in, and your brain will straighten out. If you suspect that you may be having some issues along the way, here are some thoughts on what might help.

First, you could consider seeing a doctor and getting checked out thoroughly. My Starvation Brain ended up being caused by an untreated thyroid disorder. The first two doctors I saw didn't catch it, because my TSH and T4 were normal, but finally I saw a doctor who checked my T3 (which was subterranean) and reverse T3 (which was sky-high).

Second, consider simplifying your food. Steam your cooked vegetables rather than roasting them. Let go of nuts, nut butters, and melting cheese. Use fewer ingredients and fewer condiments. Avoid eating out. Research shows that simple food allows the brain to lower our adiposity set point and accept our weight loss without fighting it with a hormonal barrage.

And finally, you could try adding some food. Research shows that protein is the most satiating macronutrient, so upping your protein (to 1.5 or 2 servings at breakfast and 1.5 servings at lunch and dinner) might really help. Starvation Brain is really hard to live with, and extended weight loss naturally and normally causes alarm in the brain, alarm that fades when we've stabilized at Maintenance. It can be tricky to know whether to tough it out and soldier on or to investigate and perhaps tweak something. Mainly, I just want you to know that you're not broken. You're not doing it wrong. You're still on the path; you're okay.

CONSIDER TREATING THE ADDICTION FIRST

If you feel like you have some form of Starvation Brain but you're most definitely not staying Bright; if you haven't been able to stay consecutively Bright for very many days at all; and, worse yet, if your Bright Days are punctuated by horrific binges, you might want to consider a significant modification to your program. I don't recommend this often, but it could be an excellent avenue to pursue if you're suffering from the trifecta: an eating disorder, a weight problem, and an as-yet-unyielding case of food addiction. Of course, definitely proceed in consultation with your doctor and your treatment team.

Remember in Chapter 3, when we were talking about how food addiction is the hardest addiction, one of the reasons being that it often creates the side effect of weight gain? And how trying to lose the weight can trigger a hormonal cascade in the brain that drives us back to addictive eating? I said that it might just be the most vicious of vicious circles to get stuck in. And the challenge is, most folks absolutely insist on addressing the weight issue with the recovery from food addiction and the treatment of the eating disorder because we are often more focused on getting the weight off than getting neutral, well, and free. That can be just fine—unless the data are in and it hasn't worked.

At that point, one way out of the vicious circle is to take a different approach and tackle the problems one at a time. Separate the treatment of the eating disorder, the food addiction, and the weight issue by leaving your weight alone at first and focusing solely on recovery. It can be significantly easier to address them one at a time and over a longer duration of recovery. After a few Bright months, once your recovery is solid, you can begin to reduce your food plan, slowly and gradually. Your single focus in the first phase is to arrest all eating disorder symptoms and get a foundation of peace and neutrality with food before you tackle any kind of weight loss.

If you have binge eating disorder or bulimia in the mix, your very first step might be to address the eating disorder portion, even before the food addiction, which might mean allowing a fourth or fifth meal if you are hungry, so long as you eat a meal and you don't binge. Legitimate physiological hunger is normal right before mealtime or bedtime, but since hunger can be a trigger for a binge, having the option to eat an additional meal, so long as you don't binge, can help keep the "Fifth Bright Line" (no bingeing, no purging) firmly in place. Once your eating disorder is in remission, you can then treat the food addiction. You should do all this on a Maintenance-level food plan, which is the amount of food your body needs to maintain, not lose, its weight.

The final phase would be to very gradually reduce the food plan so you lose weight slowly while solidly maintaining your recovery with good habits underneath you.

FOOD FREEDOM

The journey may have its ups and downs, and we each take our own unique path along the way, but at the end of the day what we're all aiming for is living in our Bright Bodies, free from food obsession and from the mindless compulsion to put food in our mouths that we don't want to be eating. What we have demonstrated in the Bright Line Eating community is that true food freedom is possible. Moreover, once you've experienced what true food freedom feels like, day after day for a week, a month, a year, it spoils you for living any other way. Nothing else remotely compares to that feeling, and you can have it. It's available here.

It's available if your Lines have been Bright from the beginning, and it's available after years of rezooming. After years of breaks, I can honestly report that today I am a free woman. Free. Not because I have less stress in my life; I don't. But because I'm not eating over the stress and the food isn't what's on my mind. This is freedom.

There is a correlation between how high you are on the Susceptibility Scale and the type of Bright Line Eating program (actions, behaviors, and attitudes) that will lead to food freedom. The higher you are on the Susceptibility Scale, the more structure, support, and automaticity you need for freedom—and the simpler your food needs to be. The lower you are on the Susceptibility Scale, the more likely you are to achieve freedom by simply picking and choosing from a few of the tools that are offered, seeing what works for you, and leaving it at that. It's not fair, but it's the truth. And no matter what, there is a path to food freedom for all of us.

AUTOMATICITY

Automaticity is, in many ways, the grease that makes the gears turn smoothly. Without it, we're relying on willpower and constantly caving. With it, we're surfing with ease, far above the Danger and Destruction Zone. Automaticity plays a role in all three aspects of our program: our food, our actions, and our support. With our food, we write down tomorrow's meals the night before in our food journal, and then the next day we focus on eating only and exactly what we wrote down. The next day we do it again. Over time, automaticity builds and, at some point, many of us find that we can stop writing down our food the night before. But here I want to point out some dangerous rocks lurking below the surf. Namely, that if you stop writing down your food during the weight-loss phase, you risk never successfully navigating the transition to Maintenance.

The explanation is simple. The key issue is this: What is our automaticity pinned to? If we notice that eating the right thing at mealtime has become completely automatic, we might feel safe to stop writing down our food the night before. But if we do that, in short order our automaticity will be pinned to following the weight-loss food plan rather than pinned to keeping the commitment to eat what we wrote down the night before.

But if we continue writing down our food, we keep the habit of consulting our food journal now and then at mealtime for a reminder of what we're supposed to eat. This allows us to add or subtract food, as needed, from our plan and stay successful when we transition to Maintenance. If our automaticity is pinned to the weight-loss food plan and we're no longer writing down our food, we're going to get wonky through that period of time when we start to add food fairly regularly.

It's really essential to have a period of time at night, after dinner, where we're thinking through what we're going to eat the next day and remembering how our food plan has changed. I have noticed that when people stop writing down their food before they are extremely settled in Maintenance, their system has resistance to adding food when it is very much needed. If and when they do add food to their plan, they're far more likely to develop a new and extremely problematic tendency to sometimes eat the new food that's been added and sometimes not. Thus begins the wonkiness, and it gets worse from there.

In short, you want to keep your automaticity pinned to eating only and exactly what you wrote down the night before, for a long, long time, until you're well along in the Maintenance dance.

COUNTING DAYS

If you're having a Bright Line Day—and maybe you did yesterday too, but maybe not—it brings up the question of whether or not to count days. If you've formally done Bright Line Eating for any stretch of time, odds are you've experienced counting days, because I typically guide people to start counting with "Day 1" on their first Bright Line Day and continue from there. But once you've had a few breaks and started over at Day 1 several times, you might find yourself asking, Why count days? There are pros and cons to both approaches.

On the one hand, starting from Day 1 is a fresh start. It feels really clean and motivating to get back on track. And then it's also really gratifying to see the passage of time as you go. Marking these days creates benchmarks to celebrate. It's been 100 Bright Line Days. It's been 10 years. These milestones, they come around.

In addition, once you've got a stack of days under your belt, counting days creates a fear of loss that can be both healthy and helpful. Human beings are very loss-averse creatures. We don't want to lose something that we currently possess. And this unique, ever-growing, and hard-won numerical day count starts to feel like an incredibly valuable possession we don't want to lose. I cannot tell you how many drinks I have *not taken* in my life solely because I didn't want to lose my years of sobriety. There have definitely been times, instances, and occasions, when if it weren't for that, I would've taken a drink. So that can be helpful too. You get enough days out and you might decide to stick with your plan just because you don't want to lose the accomplishment of those days. It may not be the most exalted motivation, but if it bolsters you in a moment of temptation, it'll do.

Now, why decide *not* to count days? Some of us make that choice. We get to a point in our journey where we decide not to count days anymore. One of the benefits of letting go of counting days is that the surrender reinforces an identity mindset. If you're just someone who does this no matter what, why count days? This also reinforces the one-day-at-a-time approach, where all the days before and all the days to come, none of them counts. What counts is today. Just for today, I put my food on the scale and I eat what I committed to eat. It can be a really helpful mental orientation.

Another helpful thing about not counting days is that it relieves the burden of trying to figure out what a Bright Line Day is, which can sometimes be tricky. You're weighing out your breakfast and you lick the yogurt spoon. Well, that wasn't weighed and measured food. And is that a break? Is that not a break? If you're counting days, you have to decide. If you're not counting days, then just rezoom, and don't do it tomorrow.

You might find that, ultimately, not counting days can be the way to define the journey that allows you to feel like you're winning. Because if you get 72 days and then go back to Day 1, and then you get 45 days and go back to Day 1, and then 93 days and go back to Day 1, at some point you will feel like asking yourself, "Wow, am I just a failure at this?" When the reality is that if you look at all those months, you've been sticking with your Bright Lines 98.6 percent of the time. Wouldn't it be nice to define the journey in a way that makes you feel like a winner and acknowledges all the Bright Line Days that you've had?

Of course, there are more nuanced ways to count days. You could count days and not go back to Day 1 if you don't have a Bright Line Day. You can just pause there and only count up the days that are Bright. You can also count all the days since you started your Bright Line Eating journey in the first place.

This is yet another place where rezooming asks you to define your journey for yourself and be honest about what works for you. You are self-responsible. Choose an approach that serves you.

A BREAK OR NOT A BREAK?

If you're going to count days, you're in the position of needing to judge whether your day was Bright or not, and that raises the question: What counts as a break? To help you make that call after a questionable situation, I have several perspectives to share with you, born of decades of hard-won experience.

First, there is a way to frame something that acknowledges that it wasn't the brightest of Bright without going back to Day 1, and that is to call it a "red flag"; in other words, a learning experience. In rezoom parlance, it's a signpost that we're quite a ways down the slope and we'd better course correct, and fast, or we'll be finding ourselves in the Danger and Destruction Zone soon.

As you decide whether to call it a break or a red flag, take a hard look at your program in general. Are you committed to your program of recovery? Working your tools? Connected to support? Or have you been in denial about the fact that you're not really engaged? If your overall program isn't strong, going back to Day 1 might be the best move because it would be a signal to start fresh and really build that strong foundation. But if you've been wholehearted about your commitment to your food recovery, then I recommend erring on the side of calling it a red flag.

You can also look at your motives in the situation in question. Was your motive to get extra food and let the hungry monster of food addiction out of the cage and gobble-gobble more, more, more? Or was your motive more innocent, where things just got away from you somehow? Life gets lifey, food gets floopy, and sometimes we just find ourselves in hard situations and slip up on the details. We are human, after all. Again, if there wasn't a part of you that decided to let it all go and indulge, I'd call it a red flag. For example, you're at a party and by mistake you take a swig of someone else's soda pop. You've already swallowed by the time you realize it's not your sparkling water. Not a break. But if you finish the glass and then drink another, that's a break.

This example highlights an important principle: *when you become aware, you become responsible*. It's simply not realistic and not kind to expect yourself to be responsible if you're not even yet aware. In my experience, though, sometimes the point of awareness isn't clear; it's extended and murky. I've spent entire restaurant meals wondering whether there was sugar in something. If it's super sweet, I stop eating immediately. But there are gray areas. I take them as learning experiences. I notice how willing I was (or wasn't) to protect my program. I get curious. I share it with someone to get it off my mind, acknowledge the red flag, and move on. Generally speaking, over the years I've become more and more convinced that the most helpful approach, if at all possible, is giving myself grace and course correcting while not going back to Day 1.

One last thought on this topic: if you're extremely high on the Susceptibility Scale, I want to point out that your deepest insides may have already determined whether it was a break or not. If you know yourself to be someone who would likely binge if you'd had a break, then if you haven't binged, perhaps that's because deep down you knew it wasn't a break. A red flag, yes. A learning experience, yes. But not a break.

EATING HEALTHY FOOD AND THE REZOOM REFRAME

To reiterate, the three shifts we need to make in order to turn the sharp spikes of the crash-and-burn cycle into the smooth sine wave of the Rezoom Reframe are: smooth off the edges, get back on the upswing faster, and raise the whole wave up to create more cushion so you never dip into the Danger and Destruction Zone.

Obviously, staying Bright is the linchpin to keeping our sine wave high, and our food choices are at the crux of that. But there's another benefit to eating according to the Bright Lines that significantly helps lift the whole sine wave. The data bear out that the way we eat is associated with less depression, less anxiety, more happiness, and more well-being.

In 2013, researchers from the University of Warwick and Dartmouth College studied the eating habits of 80,000 people in Britain.[19] They found a direct correlation between positive mental health and the consumption of fruits and vegetables. The more fruits and vegetables someone ate, the less likely they were to experience mental health challenges such as depression or anxiety. Researchers saw huge improvements in the people who increased their 3-ounce servings of vegetables from one or two to four, and in the people who increased from four servings to six. This huge linear relationship lasted up until seven servings and then it leveled out.

Another study looked at the moods of 281 young adults, average age 19.[20] What they found was that eating lots of fruits and vegetables today predicted a happy day tomorrow, and seven to eight servings of fruits and vegetables today predicted super high moods tomorrow.

The foods we eat are profoundly linked to our happiness levels. Sugar is a depressant with almost exactly the same molecular composition as alcohol. You get sugar and alcohol out of your life, your mood lifts. And this, of course, creates a positive feedback loop. The less anxious you are, the smoother the edges of your sine wave. The less depressed you are, the higher your sine wave is. And the happier you are, the better equipped you are to carry out the actions that make your whole system hum.

INNER RESISTANCE

As good as all that sounds, and as healthy as our food plan might be, we might find there are parts of us that balk at the notion of sticking with it. They might drag their feet as we try to walk through the doors of food recovery. They might keep us from "coming all the way in and sitting all the way down."

And that's okay. It's predictable and understandable.

I am going to take a moment to address a couple of the most common fears those parts might have. But a logical argument, no matter how persuasive, isn't really what they need. They need you to be curious about them and listen to them. Appendix B will be your best friend here, as it will guide you through engaging with your resistant parts in a way that will be really helpful.

That said, there are two common concerns.

Initially, the Food Indulger part of us, still very much fueled by the addiction itself and in the grip of perhaps profound dopamine downregulation, is going to balk at giving up sugar and flour. The move it will most likely make is to generate the recurring thought, *You can't do this forever. You can't imagine a world in which you'll never eat popcorn at the movies, in which you won't have cake at a wedding. You can't do Bright Line Eating.* So that Food Indulger part of you, arising from a fully hijacked nucleus accumbens, makes the argument that because you can't do this forever, you shouldn't even start doing it now.

Result: you stay stuck.

This is the trickery of the addictive mind at its most basic. It's the equivalent of a phone call saying there's $50,000 being held for you in an offshore account and all you have to do is provide your banking details and they'll wire it to you.

Don't fall for it.

It's an illusion.

Worse, it's a con.

Life is a series of nows, not one now plus a whole lot of thens. You can forget about those thens. You can do "then" whatever that Food Indulger imagines it will want then, so long as you are skillful with what you do right now.

All that counts, all that has impact, all that really matters, is that we do the next right thing, right now, today. Taking it one day at a time really is the solution. And we can comfort that part of us, that Food Indulger part that's afraid, that can't imagine that we would ever do this forever, by providing reassurance that we don't need to do this forever. We absolutely don't. We can just try it for today.

The other thing that our parts might tell us is that we'll be missing out. That Bright Line Eating will ruin our social life. That parties and holidays and traveling won't be nearly as much fun if we're not indulging.

There is a good retort to that, and in order for it to fully make sense, I need to first share some science on a phenomenon known as change blindness.

In one of the early, seminal studies of change blindness, researchers shot footage of two women having lunch. There were two camera angles, and the final video cut back and forth between the two women as they talked, as it normally would. What wasn't normal was that, unbeknownst to the viewer, the researchers changed things up in the scene with each camera cut. One woman was wearing a scarf and then she wasn't. The plates were red and then the plates were white; their arms were on the table and then, without them moving, their arms were suddenly off the table.

They played this video of what was, essentially, an impossible sequence for research participants, and the experimenters even went so far as to say to watch for changes. On average, even with the heads-up, people noticed only about 20 percent of the changes.[21]

Later research reinforced this with a famous experiment where subjects were asked to focus on how many times a basketball was being passed among people standing in a circle. Most of the subjects failed to notice a man in a gorilla suit who walked into the middle of the circle, beat his chest, and then walked off the screen.[22] This phenomenon is related to change blindness. It's called inattentional blindness; we're essentially blind to something unless we're explicitly paying attention to it.

It works in real life too. Studies have been done showing that the majority of people don't even notice if the person they just started talking to suddenly becomes a different person.[23] The study has been performed in lots of ways; for example, with a clerk behind a desk who bends out of sight to get some papers and when they straighten up, they've done a quick switch with someone who was crouched behind the desk—with a different color shirt, different height, everything. It's beyond mind-blowing, but more often than not, *people don't even notice the change.* Not because they're not smart—the study was done at Harvard. It is just human nature.

There is an extremely valuable point here. In any given moment we're absorbing only a tiny fraction of what's going on around us. We're not noticing, as we sit here, the pressure of the chair against the backs of our thighs, and we're not noticing the feeling of our feet in our socks. Another way of saying this is that we are all "missing out" on so much, all the time.

This is helpful to know as you think about how to respond to that part of you that's likely to say or feel at some point, *But if I give up sugar and flour, won't I be missing out? If my friends go out drinking, won't I be missing out? If we're having a pizza party at work, won't I be missing out? If I'm going to France and not having a croissant, won't I be missing out?*

Since we're only ever taking in a very tiny fraction of being alive in terms of our human interactions, surroundings, and experiences, the reality is that you'll always and forever only be experiencing a sliver of what was available to be experienced during those moments.

With Bright Line Eating, you shift from experiencing *this* subset of what's available to *that* subset of what's available. It's like shifting your awareness from Focus A to Focus B. Yes, you're going to be experiencing less in the food and alcohol realm, for sure. I'm not going to lie there—it's true and it's a loss. But that's going to open up some space for you to experience an equivalent amount more in other realms—in terms of art, architecture, relationships, conversation, and all the rest. Maybe you'll end up having an incredible conversation because you're not focused on silently debating whether to order dessert. You'll notice so much more of what's going on around you because you're not fixated on food. You'll get to go for a gorgeous hike with friends because you have energy and your joints don't hurt anymore.

Definitely bring compassion to that part of you that's worried, but I want your Authentic Self to internalize that what you're doing is trading in the experience of one set of things (alcohol and excess food) for the experience of a different set of things. And I would argue it is a better set of things that will bring you lasting pleasure.

All that said, if you can still feel a part of yourself bristling at these arguments, refusing to adopt these alternate perspectives, or maybe even standing in the corner, arms crossed, with a defiant sneer, you might very well have a strong Rebel part in play. I certainly did until I began working with Everett. If you resist following rules, even the ones that can dramatically improve and perhaps even save your life, this is a great opportunity to meet the part of you that likes to push back.

THE REBEL PART

If you are a person with a strong Food Controller, you may have found the structure and precision of Bright Line Eating to be comforting and even exciting once you realized the results you were getting. People with strong controlling parts frequently say that all they needed to know was what to do; they follow the program exactly as laid out, and soon they are in their Bright Bodies and their lives have been completely transformed. But many of us have parts that resist structure and control, and that brings us to the Rebel.

If you have a strong Rebel part, you are probably very aware of what you might think of as a rebellious streak. People who have strong Rebels tend to take pride in the fact that they don't go with the crowd, and it becomes a part of their identity.

It's easy to see if you have a Rebel part. Just think about the parts of your program that you won't do as prescribed. Do you have issues around writing down your food and committing it to someone? How about issues around eating exactly what you've committed? Instead, do you want to choose your foods as you make your meals? How about weighing your food? Do you resist being exact in your weights? Do you think it doesn't matter if you weigh your vegetables because they don't add much to total calories? How about eating between meals? Have you created your own rules around that? Does the fact that Bright Line Eating is so controlled make you angry? Do you have a belief that restriction is damaging? How about external support? Do you resist reaching out? Do you think that you know a better way? These are all signs you might have a Rebel part interfering with your program.

Having a strong Rebel might look like long stretches of squeaky clean Bright Lines and then mysteriously not being willing to do the program at all or switching back and forth. Rebel parts tend to be angry. Think about what type of life circumstances create a Rebel; Bright Line Eating can feel like the overly controlled and restrictive environment of our upbringing. There is one big difference, though, which is that you are choosing Bright Line Eating. It is not being forced on you by an external entity. There are no Bright Line Eating police, and you are welcome to modify Bright Line Eating in any way that you like. In this chapter there is a section on the 4 Questions and how to use them to customize Bright Line Eating in a way that works for you.

But what do you do if you have a strong Rebel interfering in your program? First off, realize that this part is trying to help you. It is really worried that something bad will happen if you conform. You could start with some inner dialogue or some journaling where you explain to the Rebel that no one is forcing you to do Bright Line Eating, and in fact, you've done a lot of research and are choosing this for your health. What might be better to rebel against is the Global Industrial Diet, which is trying to control you and addict you to its hyperpalatable foods. Sometimes something this simple is enough to get the Rebel under control. See other tools to really go in depth and discover your Rebel in Appendix B.

Lastly, *surrender* is a magical word in Bright Line Eating. It describes what happens when we have no resistance to doing the plan as described. No resistance to committing food. No resistance to weighing and measuring. No resistance to having BLE buddies and reaching out for and providing support. The weight melts off us. The food becomes neutral and we start to feel real freedom. We settle into a Bright Body and maintain it with ease. Surrender is the experience of quieting your Rebel.

CHAPTER 6

ACTIONS

As I was outlining the Rezoom System in my mind for the first time, I wrangled with the word *actions* a lot. I could have chosen *behaviors*, or *habits*, or *automaticity*. But when we're in crisis, we don't have control over whether or not we have a habit, and we don't have control over whether or not that habit feels automatic. We do, however, have control over taking one tiny action.

Actions are very small, manageable things that we can do right now, in this moment, to get us into rezoom mode. When we're following the Bright Line Eating plan, our actions, performed faithfully over time, will turn into habits, and then those habits will become automatic. Automaticity is achieved when we execute our actions without any particular effort, willpower, or cognitive load.

In terms of automaticity with actions, the main lesson is that you need to layer in new actions *gradually* in order to manage the large cognitive load brought on by introducing a new behavior, to allow time for each of them to develop into habits that don't require as much willpower, planning, or thought.

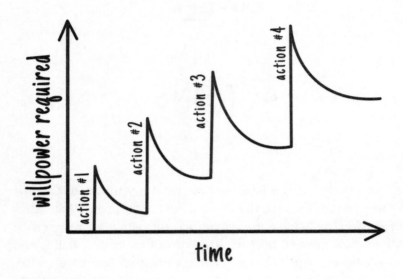

With any given action that you introduce, day after day, the amount of willpower required to do it will go down and down. And then, after a period of time, you can add in a second action. If you try to add them all at the same time, you'll overwhelm the system and not be able to stick with it.

The most important actions at first are just writing down your food the night before and then eating only and exactly that. Then you'll want to add in one of the actions we're about to discuss in this chapter. And then another. And then, perhaps, another.

I've often wondered how many habits are enough, and when I was creating the Reboot Rezoom course, there was a moment when I got an insight into the answer. Each week, to create the talking points for the videos I was going to shoot for the course, I would get together with all the Bright Line Eating coaches to brainstorm. When we got to the sections on actions that covered the morning and evening routines, I took a poll. I asked each of them to share what actions their morning and evening routines consisted of. The range of answers was incredible. While we all stayed deeply supported and connected within the Bright Line

Eating community, there was tremendous variation, including everything from a three-hour extended habit stack (which we will discuss soon) to hardly any morning routine at all. It goes back to that balance point—find what works for you.

When we're in a lapse mode and wanting to shift into the upswing of rezoom mode, we need to focus on the tiny actions we can do right now to turn it around. In Bright Line Eating, we say that we are not called to be perfect; we are called to be unstoppable. We *have* to be unstoppable because we're facing foods that are as addictive as cocaine, cues to indulge all around us, and brains that are way more vulnerable than average. And while the overall goal is to *not eat addictively*, what I've learned is that when you're starting to lapse, the food is actually usually the last out, meaning it's the other components of the framework—the actions and support—that start to slip first. If you start to notice your actions and your support slipping, it's a clue that your food is about to slip. Developing this awareness is part of crafting a gentler ride, because as you become mindful that your actions and support are sliding, you can pull yourself up into rezoom mode much faster, before you're breaking your Bright Lines. Knowledge is power.

ACTIONS AND IDENTITY

In James Clear's number-one *New York Times* best-selling book *Atomic Habits*, a favorite in the Bright Line Eating community, he talks about why sustained behavior change is so hard, and he points out that people often come at it from the wrong direction. He presents the following schematic, showing the three levels at which change can take place. He describes that we can go from the outside in, or from the inside out.

THREE LAYERS OF BEHAVIOR CHANGE

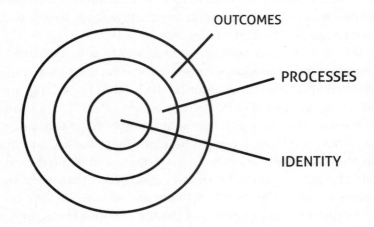

At the center is identity. In the middle is process. And on the outside are outcomes. A lot of people orient their Bright Line Eating journey in terms of outcomes. They want to lose 20 pounds, or 200. They want to fit into a particular outfit, suit, or dress by the time their daughter gets married. They want to bring their blood sugar down so they won't have to start taking the insulin their doctor threatened them with.

The challenge is that long-term change isn't sustained when we focus on the outside and move our way in. That's the wrong direction. It's sustained when we focus on the center first, at the level of identity, meaning what we believe about ourselves.

The key to long-term, sustained behavior change is to focus on building a new identity first, then considering the process—the actions, habits, or systems that will get us where we want to go—and then mostly letting the outcomes take care of themselves. The magical thing is that when we make the inner two layers our focus, the outcomes naturally follow.

When I'm coaching, I can often tell in two minutes whether I'm coaching someone who is focused on building a new identity or focused on achieving some particular outcome. If they're primarily outcome focused, they're likely to be talking about their weight loss with impatience and dissatisfaction, even if their weight loss is continuing right on schedule. If they have reached their Bright Body but did it with an outcome focus, odds are they're struggling now because, without a solid identity to make it clear that nothing really ends or changes in Maintenance, they start breaking their Lines as soon as the outcome is reached. In contrast, folks who are identity focused tend to be in it for the long haul, and they're not in a rush. Their Lines stay Bright during weight loss and equally Bright during Maintenance. They're focused on how grateful they are for their Bright Transformation.

From my perspective, there simply is no overemphasizing how pivotal the identity piece is. And the good news is, a new identity isn't as hard to build as you might think.

James Clear gives the formula, right there in Chapter 2 of *Atomic Habits*. It's a simple, two-step process:

1. Decide the type of person you want to be.

2. Prove it to yourself with small wins.

If you want freedom from cravings, a lifetime of enjoying your Bright Body, plus peace and serenity with food—in short, if you want your life back or maybe a better life than you've ever had—the identity to adopt is someone who just follows the friggin' plan. Bright Line Eating is a process that also provides an identity. "I am a Bright Lifer. I am someone who does Bright Line Eating." That's who you want to become.

How do you do that?

You write down what you're going to eat tomorrow. When tomorrow dawns, for breakfast, you eat only and exactly what you wrote down. For lunch, you eat only and exactly what you wrote down. And for dinner, you eat only and exactly what you wrote down. Those small actions, day in and day out, build your identity. You're sticking with the plan. You do Bright Line Eating.

Each Bright meal, each new action practiced faithfully, at the same time each day, in service of your budding automaticity, and each log-in to the Bright Line Eating community proves to yourself who you are. Before long, you'll find that being someone who does Bright Line Eating has become part and parcel of your whole life, and you'll know that to be true about yourself at a very deep level.

TAKING IT FURTHER

I love James Clear's identity framework. It's brilliant. And, from a Bright Line Eating perspective, we can add a little twist to bring it to the next level. Here's the thing: when it comes to that middle ring of *process*, Bright Line Eating is incredible. It's highly structured, taking participants step-by-step from not knowing anything to having a spectacular level of mastery, automaticity, and mind-blowing results. But the first step on the journey isn't—and can't be—having a fully built Bright Identity. The *first step* is simply committing to the process wholeheartedly. JFTFP. Just follow the friggin' plan.

Then, after we commit, an amazing thing happens: Self-Perception Theory kicks in. This is from Daryl Bem of Cornell University, who proposed in 1972 that human beings learn who they are—their attitudes, beliefs, desires, and even their core character—by observing their own behavior. So as we accumulate those daily wins through committing to the process, we start to grow our identity as someone who is committed to the process. A Bright Lifer, through and through. This is how we can go from being someone who could never imagine not eating sugar and flour for a single day to becoming someone who really doesn't mind the thought of not eating sugar and flour forever because our Bright Identity is so strong.

This also means bringing process to the forefront of our attention and allowing outcomes to recede. At the beginning, whatever our ideal outcome is, whether it's to lose 100 pounds by our birthday next year or to get off those statins, we're going to sell ourself short if we measure success solely by that outcome. We could follow the system to a tee, which is the biggest win there is, and fall short of that target number by two pounds and end up feeling like a failure, which would be tragic.

So hold the outcomes very loosely and instead surrender to the process. In the fullness of time, we're likely to find that our Bright Identity rewards us in ways that we can't yet imagine—physically, mentally, spiritually, and emotionally. As that happens, our notion of "outcomes" will expand beyond the beyond.

In a nutshell, it goes like this. We start by committing to the process—JFTFP, one day at a time. Gradually, our Bright Identity grows, from nothing at first to a solid steel core that straightens our spine and lifts us up in everything we do. And the outcomes, if held gently at first, will, over time, expand as our universe grows and the Non-Scale Victories accumulate. Here's what that looks like in a visual:

Three Layers of Behavior Change

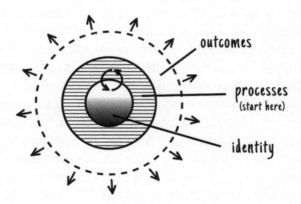

outcomes

processes
(start here)

identity

ACTIONS, FEELINGS, THOUGHTS

In psychology, a body of research looked at the relationships among our actions, our feelings, and our thoughts, and what it found was that they all influence each other bidirectionally. Our actions impact our feelings, and our feelings impact our actions. Our feelings impact our thoughts, and our thoughts impact our feelings. Bidirectional relationships all around.

Then, over the next decade or so, that research went deeper and found that the most powerful directionality is from actions to thoughts and feelings, meaning that our actions strongly influence what we think and how we feel.

Action → → → → Thoughts & Feelings

Furthermore, if you look at the question of volition, choice, will, or influence in terms of what we can control, our actions are the things that we can exert the most direct control over. If you go to 12-Step meetings, you'll often hear people say you can't think your way into right action, but you can act your way into right thinking. Actions are the most powerful lever.

If we turn our attention to the things that we can change with our actions, like going to bed early, meditating, eating a glorious Bright meal, and making a phone call to a Bright friend or buddy, and then we look at the impact of now being in a world in which we've gotten a good night's sleep, meditated, eaten a Bright meal, and been in contact with a friend, we see how that new environment has such a powerful impact on our well-being. Our thoughts and feelings will be drastically different in that new reality. When we do different, we *are* different.

The longer I travel on this recovery journey, the more I choose to focus on my actions, almost to the exclusion of all else. I care how my thinking is and I care how my feelings are, but I know that the driver of my recovery is my actions, and this is why my various measuring and monitoring tools of journals and calendars and nightly checklists are so powerful for me. I'm measuring what I'm seeking to control and exert influence over because it's through changing my actions that I can change my thoughts and feelings and really up-level my whole life.

The goal is to reach a state where no matter how outrageous the circumstances of our life, no matter how much stress, emotional turmoil, or strain we're experiencing, our brain never suggests that eating over it might be a good idea. We never consider doing the thing that used to seem like it would solve and soothe but that always actually opened a chasm that took days, weeks, or months to climb out from. The options that do pop into our mind now are other things, like, *Maybe I should go to bed early, or have a good cry, or do some food prep so my next meal is all ready for me when it's time to eat.*

When I was pregnant with my twins, my due date was August 16. On April 25, I went into labor, was admitted to the hospital, and was told: You're here for the duration. And your twins have a 4 percent chance of both surviving and being healthy. All through that time, I just weighed and measured the next meal and took care of my emotional needs by leaning on family and friends. My brain never suggested to me that I should eat something different from my plan. Did staying calm and strong through that time and *not* eating a lot of unhealthy foods help? I'll never know, but today those twins are both healthy teenagers, and I'm so glad I nourished myself—and them—well in those days before they were born weighing under a pound and a half each.

No matter the circumstances, I promise, it's possible. And that is what I want for you: a brain that's neutral and steady and detached from life's most painful fluctuations.

The more we reinforce to our Indulger that "treats" are *not* what to expect, the more we will create a brain that never proposes otherwise, because it knows that it would be futile since that's not how this captain runs the ship.

And that's when you have long-term peace. That's what you're in the game for—to not give addictive foods any more of yourself, your heart, your time, or your precious mental resources. It's not worth it. The peace is better.

DAILY RITUALS

There are a host of actions that can bolster our food recovery program, and the core set of actions, collectively, make up our daily rituals. They are the ropes that guide us from place to place through a Bright Day. Sometimes keeping our Lines Bright can be an hour-to-hour achievement. These rituals will both give you a soft place to land and bolster the next part of your day. I want to restore your sense of sovereignty over your body, your behaviors, and your choices. Rituals help to do that by healing your brain, reinvigorating your sense of control, and setting you up for success.

THE HABIT STACK

The habit stack was first created by Stanford social scientist BJ Fogg in his book *Tiny Habits* and then further popularized by James Clear. It is the foundation of the Bright Line morning and evening rituals. A habit stack is a series of habits that you perform in the same way, every time, one after the other, so that completing one action is the cue to do the next action. It's a series of dominoes, where one falls and trips the next one. You can set the whole thing in motion with very little effort, and before you know it, you're out the other end, having achieved more productive self-care in a short span of time than perhaps you used to achieve all day.

I used to have a morning routine habit stack beginning when my alarm went off, which would trigger me to get out of bed, which then triggered me to stretch and drop down on my knees to pray. From there I'd stand and walk to the bathroom and sit down, which was a cue to reach for my inspirational book, read a passage, and deeply ponder it. Standing from there would trigger me to reach for my tape measure, measure my waist, and then step on the scale. (I don't weigh myself daily anymore—I'm back to weekly—but during this stretch of time, I did.)

From there I'd take my thyroid medicine and head downstairs to my office to sit and meditate. When the alarm went off signaling that it was over, I would put on my exercise clothes and go around the corner to my little home gym area and do a workout.

Then I'd come out from the gym area, make myself a cup of black coffee and my breakfast just as the kids would be coming downstairs, and I'd get them all ready and on the bus to school. That would trigger me to go back into my office to do the Bright Lifers Accountability Call. And when the Accountability Call was over, it would be my cue to go upstairs and take a shower, make my bed, and get dressed for the day.

That right there was a three-and-a-half-hour regimen that I performed just about every day in the same way, with each action triggering me to perform the next action because I did them in the same order, in the same way, every time. My habit stacks tend to be on the long side. But effective habit stacks can also be quite short and simple. You might already have a habit stack for brushing your teeth. If, for example, you brush and floss and use mouthwash, that's an example of a mini habit stack—a few actions that you perform, one after the other in the same way, every day. You probably have a habit stack for getting dressed, where you put on the same article of clothing first, and then the next and the next.

What's great about a habit stack is that it can get really wired in, becoming truly automatic, and you can get a tremendous amount done using very little willpower and few cognitive reserves. It's an amazing way to be outrageously productive. In order to achieve that, though, you have to be consistent. There's a huge difference between meditating every day for a week at haphazard times and meditating every day for a week at the same time triggered by the same specific cue. As you build these little habit stacks of actions, I want you to consider that the more you can do them the same way every day, the more you will be investing in a free tomorrow. You have the motivation today, so set it all up so that it doesn't matter whether you feel motivated tomorrow.

Another huge benefit of a habit stack is that, as you move forward in life and you come across something you really want to do or accomplish—say, learn Italian by spending 20 minutes a day with an app—if you already have a habit stack in place, all you have to do is slide those 20 minutes into your habit stack and you'll be cued to do it every day. In this way and for this reason, people with existing habit stacks are way more successful at long-term behavior change of all sorts.

Beyond that, it can be a great way to set up times of your day when you may have been vulnerable to triggers in the past. If you have found that you kind of float between the end of your workday and bedtime, leaving you vulnerable to a slew of impulses, creating a habit stack for that part of your day might be hugely beneficial. Something that moves you from specific place to specific place with a clear, positive action attached. An example might be, "I go down to the parking lot after work and get my yoga bag out of the trunk." (This assumes you are on Maintenance and have added exercise back into your life.) "Seeing it on the seat beside me reinforces that I am heading to a class I enjoy. After class, I go straight home to cook a Bright Line meal. While dinner cooks, I unpack my wet clothes and put them right in the wash and repack my yoga bag and put it by the door for tomorrow. I watch one hour of TV, and then I get ready for bed and wind down with a book that inspires me." To that you could add additional bedtime routines—perhaps journaling or meditating or writing a gratitude list.

Having a preplanned routine of actions that you have chosen from your Authentic Self can help you move through wobbly hours of vulnerability. Eventually this stack just becomes what you do without even thinking about it.

There is an enormous range in the scope and breadth of actions that successful Bright Lifers build into their morning and evening routines. Some, like me, have elaborate habit stacks that take a long time to execute. Others have much briefer routines. Some journal in the morning, some in the evening, and others not at all. What's common among us is that we prioritize self-care and ritualize it into routines that take the load off willpower and bolster our commitment to living Bright each day.

MORNING ROUTINES

From the moment we return to consciousness in the morning, our first few choices will set the tone for our day.

A long time ago, I built the habit of starting each and every day by taking a moment to say thank you for the day I'm about to receive. I slide out of bed and drop down to my knees in full prostration, also known as child's pose, nose to the ground. I know every day is a blessing to all of us, but I also know that I engaged in some behaviors when I was using drugs that I am truly lucky to have survived. I thank God for every chance I get to do things differently. Then I set my intention to have a Bright Day, to be of service today, and I ask for God's help to do just that.

Now, let me just emphasize here that there is absolutely no requirement in Bright Line Eating that anybody believe or do any specific things when it comes to spirituality or religion. That's entirely up to you. Nor will it determine your success or failure with rezooming. But being intentional about how you spend the first moments of your day is worthwhile because it sets the tone.

The rest of the morning routine continues from there and could include some specific components you might want to con-sider adding in, if you don't do them already. But before we dive in, I do want to reiterate that there's only so much you can change at one given time and expect it to hold because it takes willpower to do these things before they become automatic. And willpower is a finite resource. That means you might be in a state right now of being months away from your ideal morning habit stack, and that's okay.

Regardless, the important thing is to become the equivalent of a lifelong learner when it comes to the morning routine and to develop the identity of someone who is always scanning, looking for ways to tweak and improve it. Expect it to change, morph, and evolve. For example, sometimes I have exercise in my morn-ing routine, but sometimes I'm just in daily minimalist mode and focused on keeping my Lines Bright and exercise comes out of there. Sometimes I'm on caffeine and making a cup of black coffee is part of my morning routine, but sometimes I'm off caffeine and that's out of there.

The morning routine is fluid. It changes. But the important thing is to develop the identity of someone who's always scanning, always considering, always looking for improvements. Remember: you are flying the plane—keep checking the instrument panel! Don't go on autopilot if you are gliding down toward the Danger and Destruction Zone.

Right now, I invite you to consider your morning routine and see if you can make it a notch better, a notch more streamlined, a notch more helpful, a notch in the direction you want to go in. And if you don't have a morning routine much beyond throwing on clothes and rushing out the door, you have a huge opportunity to up-level your life, and it starts now.

INSPIRATIONAL READING

When I first got clean and sober from drugs, I was told to sit quietly and read a daily meditation book every morning. So I did— while I chain-smoked several cigarettes and drank super-sweet, ultra-creamy coffee. The practice has come a long way since then, but sitting quietly and reflecting on something spiritual each morning (but *without* the coffee and cigarettes) is still an essential cornerstone for me.

On the Rezoom website there are a host of resources, and among them you can find a list of daily readers I recommend at https://RezoomBook.com, but any positive, uplifting daily meditation book will do. If you have a religious practice where you are enjoined by your faith to read some scripture morning and night, beautiful. If not, and you've never anchored your morning with a page from a daily meditation reader, simply check out the list of resources and pick one that calls to you.

I predict you'll find that this simple action changes the whole day, and the reason is that it shifts activity in the brain. The part of the brain that is pulled by addictive food is small. It is essentially trapped in a tiny chemical prison, focus down, just circling around one thing over and over for eternity. When we start each day by introducing a big thought, it widens our focus right off the bat and stimulates activity in higher centers of the brain. That pulls us out of ourselves and reminds us of the vastness of the universe and our mysteriously perfect place in it.

MAKING THE BED

I am a big fan of making my bed every day, and making it *well*. Crisp lines. Taut sheets. I invite you to become a devotee of this practice too. Perhaps that seems obvious to you—perhaps that's how you've been making your bed for decades—but I have to say that when I suggest this in my Boot Camps, I sometimes get a strong response. This could be because we are a community of formerly hungover people, and whether it was from sugar or alcohol, most of us gave our bad habits free rein after dark—thus making for awful mornings. So we need to be reminded to start making our beds. When we do, we are starting the day with an act of respect for ourselves and our home that immediately says to our brains, "I am someone who accomplishes tasks and prioritizes taking exceptional care of myself." It might sound small, but it is the first brick in the foundation of your day.

MEDITATION

Neuroscientific research has shown that the right prefrontal cortex is the seat of depression and foul moods and the left prefrontal cortex is the seat of peace and ease and bliss and happiness. And if you look at the minds of consistent meditators, they show a dramatic shift in activation, overall, from the right prefrontal cortex to the left. Moreover, research shows that participants can create that shift in as little as 10 to 15 minutes of meditation a day over a stretch of eight to ten weeks.[24] It doesn't take long to actually rewire your brain to produce more happiness on a consistent basis just by using meditation.

Meditation also creates a lot of emotional stability, which for many of us is really helpful. Being high on the Susceptibility Scale means I have a predisposition to addiction, and two of the traits correlated with addiction are impulsivity and extra heightened sensitivity. Meditation creates the emotional stability that helps me remember that what other people do isn't generally about me—it's about *them*.

But in our rezoom context, ultimately the reason to meditate is that it will raise the curve. Meditation is one of the key behaviors that creates the cushion and raises our cycles above the Danger and Destruction Zone—that's the shift from right to left prefrontal cortex at work. Meditation also smooths off the edges. It builds in a pause where we can practice some self-compassion and not experience any given moment as a sharp emergency. And it helps with the third shift too—pulling out of a downslide and getting on the upswing much faster. When we meditate regularly, we build in time to assess our life and our program and we are far more likely to notice when we're on a slippery slope. From a rezoom perspective, meditation delivers the trifecta. It truly is foundational.

Despite all the enormous benefits of meditation, you might find the thought of starting a regular meditation practice daunting. I know I did. For years upon years, I had a desire in the back of my mind to start meditating, but I procrastinated and put it off—until one of my mentors showed me a way of thinking about meditation that made it seem less scary. She told me that the key to meditating is to simply sit still. She said, "I don't care if you cross your legs or sit in a chair or sit on the couch or stand on your head, just don't do anything. No movement. No activity. No distractions. Nothing. For thirty minutes."

Finally, I was willing. She told me to set a timer and just sit there. So I did. And for many years, my meditation practice just consisted of quiet time. I didn't make any real effort to regulate what I was doing during those 30 minutes other than keeping myself physically still.

The benefit I got from setting aside that time, almost immediately, was a deep sense of comfort in my own skin. I can be at peace with myself even if I feel awful, if I feel sick, if I feel angry, if I feel really hungry, or if I'm having a food thought or a craving or an obsession. I can sit with those feelings and just let them be. And that is something I most definitely could not do when I first started to meditate. From my subsequent years of teaching Bright

Line Eating, I now think meditation is the most important action we can take.

The key benefit for people like me, who are trying to live lives free from the tyranny of addiction, is just learning to develop a pause between all the stimuli in our environment and our response to them. So much of life's chaos comes from reactivity, from allowing our amygdala, the core fight-or-flight part of our brains, to trigger a response before we can catch our breath and get more information. Maybe the guy meant to cut you off, or maybe—let's take a pause and come around the parking lot one more time—it's actually a woman trying to hand a banana to the child in the back seat with one hand and who is now mouthing, "I'm sorry," at you through her windshield. Aren't you glad you didn't start honking and cursing? Learning to lengthen and strengthen that pause is a huge gift. It will give you a way to regulate your emotions and thoughts before you run to your food habit for comfort. It's a respite.

The number one barrier that I think keeps most people from meditating is what yogis call monkey mind: the way our thoughts pinball from one thing to the next ad infinitum. It's uncomfortable to meditate, especially if you go in with any kind of expectation of trying to quiet or still your mind or watch your breath. Because the reality is that our thought life is really distracting and chaotic. So don't worry about what your head's doing. Expect the monkey mind. In fact, invite it into the process. If you expect that your thoughts are going to bebop around, it can become a source of fascination and curiosity. *Where are my thoughts going to go? What's going to pop into my head this time?* Resolve to be curious.

The monkey mind can be pretty magical. It's one of the key ways I get to experience dancing with the universe in this mystery of life. What shows up in my morning meditation is a window into what matters, what I care about, what needs to get unraveled. Sometimes someone I haven't thought about in years will pop into my head. And then they call the next day or I call them, and it turns out they really needed to hear from me for some reason.

If I have a course to create, I make sure that I meditate, deeply and for longer, because that's the space where my monkey mind will sort out what needs to go into the content, taking this gnarly ball of yarn that is my thought life and unraveling it.

If monkey mind has been a barrier that's prevented you from creating a regular meditation practice, I invite you to consider flipping that around. Get excited and curious about it, and log it as a win if you sit there and do the meditation at all.

THE CUE TO MEDITATE

The goal right now is to make your practice automatic. Otherwise, trying to meditate can be a big willpower drain if you find you have a loop of *I should meditate, I should meditate, I should meditate* running in the background.

One of the best ways to not have that is to meditate first thing in the morning. Now, if you have a feeling that a different time of day, whether it's late morning or afternoon or evening or right before bed, is your best time to meditate and it's working for you, then by all means do that. Do what works for you.

The piercing question I want you to ask yourself, though, is: Are you *actually* doing that? Because if you have it in your head that you should be meditating in the evening and you're not doing it, then it's not working for you. Getting it tucked away first thing in the morning might be a better strategy, in part because mornings are the time of day over which people generally have the most control.

When we're traveling or when people are visiting, as soon we get out of those early morning hours, the day gallops away and it's much harder to predict what's going to happen. Rarely do we get an invitation to do something social at 7:00 A.M. But the invitations to do things with other people that stretch into the evening and butt up against bedtime and wreak havoc with the evening routine are frequent.

For that reason, one of my key strategies to balancing a morning and an evening routine is to stack as much as possible into the morning routine. What's your cue that precedes meditation? What's the trigger in that habit stack? What is the antecedent? I want you to have that clearly defined, because it is the domino that's going to trip that meditation domino to fall over. The more you can make that a salient, predictable cue, the better.

BFF

No, we are not sixth-grade girls and going to be best friends forever. This is an acronym Everett came up with that stands for: Breathe, Feel your body, Find your feet. When you feel yourself starting to get overwhelmed or dysregulated, take a few deep breaths, drop into your body, notice and observe how it feels, and find the part of you that is connected to the earth—be it your feet or your seat—and dial into that sense of groundedness.

Unlike your mediation practice, you can do this at any time, anywhere you need to take a breath and ground yourself. Whenever you need to hit the pause button, practice BFF and you'll increase your connection to your body and boost your parasympathetic nervous system, that calm-and-restore part of yourself.

People who come to this work tend to have a history of eating over their emotions. But if we learn to tune in to our body during an emotion, really sitting inside our own body, watching where that emotion is and where we're feeling it in our body and staying present with it, the feeling dissipates within one to two minutes. The feeling might come back later, usually triggered by thoughts, but then we can drop back into our body again, be present with the pure feeling, and watch it dissolve. It's a powerful practice that will truly benefit anyone with a lifetime of emotional eating habits to overcome.

COMMITTING

In Bright Line Eating, we write down what we intend to eat the next day and then, when those meals arrive, we eat only and exactly that. But the key intermediary step is taking that intended food plan, whatever we've written down, and committing it.

Now, there are lots of different ways you could do that. You could do it with someone who supports you unidirectionally; that person would be called a guide in Bright Line Eating and a sponsor in 12-Step programs.

You → → → → Guide/Sponsor

Your guide (or sponsor) would be someone whom you call every day, usually at a specific time, and tell them what you're going to eat for either that day or the next day, and go over the other things that might be going on in your life. It can be hugely helpful.

Or you could have a bidirectional commitment relationship, and we call that a buddy. You commit your food to them, and they commit their food to you, bidirectionally.

You → → → → Buddy

Buddy → → → → You

You can also commit your food to a group. Many people in Bright Line Eating belong to small groups, whether online or through one of the various apps people use for connecting, and you could commit your food there. Or you could commit it in the Bright Line Eating Online Support Community. It's a perfectly fine thing to commit your food publicly to a large group like that.

You can do it in the evening, right after you write down your plan for the next day, or you can do it the following morning before your day gets going. Whichever you pick, always do it the same way consistently, though I would suggest that you not use multiple methods. The reason is this: if you commit by telling a buddy *and* posting it online, then if one day you only manage to commit in one of those places, you might feel half-committed. You don't want to put yourself in that situation.

When I was first recovering from food addiction, I committed my food every single day for a long stretch of time. I usually don't do it anymore unless I need some extra support for a while. You'll find that, most likely, you won't need to do it forever. But be careful thinking that you're there too soon. It took me many months to get to a place where it felt wise to stop committing my food. And as for writing it down the night before, I continued doing that for five full years. Not five months—five years. So I encourage you to find a way to commit, start doing it, make it a habit, and watch what happens. It's going to serve you really well.

IF IT ISN'T

Not to sound like I am contradicting myself, but to paraphrase Carl Jung, healing comes in embracing paradox, so here goes: stop doing it if it's not working. This means if you're writing down your food and committing it to someone but frequently breaking your commitment and eating something else, then committing your food to that person is no longer helpful because you're actually reinforcing the action of not following through. Each time you commit and then deviate, it creates yet another opportunity for you to break your integrity. Yet another opportunity for you to witness letting yourself and someone else down.

As soon as you've experienced a few times where you've committed in a particular way and noticed that having made that commitment doesn't make you feel super beholden, then it's not working and you should stop. Do not put yourself in the position of watching yourself be unfaithful over and over and over again.

When we commit, it only works if we grant authority to that commitment structure. The only way we know we're actually giving it authority is if it's holding us in a state where we follow through.

This goes for taking someone else's food commitment as well. If they keep breaking their Lines and not eating what they committed, you're not doing them any favors by continuing to take their food commitment.

In sum, I cannot emphasize enough how the morning routine has been the foundation for me. There's a Yiddish saying: "Lose an hour in the morning, chase it all day." If I wake up late or I sleep in and I don't do my morning routine, I have this feeling all day long that I'm behind, that I'm trying to catch up. And that creates a nagging, recurring thought: *Should I try to find a time to squeeze in my meditation, or should I just let it go?* Or *I need to work out* or *Shoot, I didn't do my reading,* and that thought loop is incredibly willpower depleting. It's the worst way to go through the day.

So, as you rezoom, the first thing I would invest in is a simple, basic morning habit stack that will set you up for success all day long.

EVENING ROUTINE

The evening routine encompasses looking backward on the day, our tracking, our accountability, *and* all the actions that involve looking forward to the next day. Because in my world, a Bright Day begins at sunset the night before, conceptually speaking. I know that we sometimes think of the new day as beginning at dawn, or perhaps at midnight, but I propose that in terms of Bright rhythms, the day begins at sunset. Meaning that by the time you wake up the next morning, you are already the recipient of a set of actions you took the night before that set you up to have a good day, in terms of the sleep you got; the food plan you thought through, wrote down, and committed; and the habit stacks you have in place to be executed.

If you arrive in your morning without the things you need to feel calm and empowered, then you're already behind the eight ball, which sets you up to carry an emotional and self-regulatory load that will keep you in a precarious position and vulnerable to the Willpower Gap. If you wake up late, feel groggy, over-caffeinate, get stuck in traffic, arrive without the report you stayed up late finishing, and get scolded, you could find yourself overwhelmed by a whole host of feelings you want to numb out—before lunch.

This is why the mother of the morning routine is the evening routine. You can't give birth to a good morning routine if you haven't done your evening routine on time and faithfully. Bright

Line Living does involve a certain amount of discipline at night, to shut down the day in a way that is a gift to the future you the next morning.

In the same way that I feel qualified to teach about food struggles because I have struggled with my food, when it comes to the evening routine, it's the same drill. I am not someone who easily shuts down the day and goes to bed at the right time. I'm a night owl by constitution, and I have put a lot of work into nailing my evening routine so I can wake up on time the next morning and have a solid start to my day.

This is where the habit stack comes back in. There are actions I need to take in the evening to shut down my household. First I shut down my kitchen. Then there are actions I need to take in my office and at my computer to help me be accountable to the various systems that I've set up to help me. And then there are things that I do in my bedroom and bathroom to put my personal day to bed.

For years I found myself going from one room to the next and then back until I realized that, if I'm explicit about the things I need to do in each location every night to shut down my life successfully, I can create little habit stacks *room by room* so that finishing in one room becomes the cue to head to the next room and start the next mini-sequence. Now I do them in the same way every time, which is the best way to set up routines that become automatic.

The evening routine begins by getting out that food journal and making that list of what you plan to eat the next day. I recommend doing it after dinner but before any relaxation activities. This is when you'll be the freshest.

Then, if you are an evening committer, commit your food plan for the following day. After you do, you'll relax, knowing the bulk of the next day is taken care of. Your only task for the next day will be to eat only and exactly what you've written down. That's it. No decisions to make in the moment, no negotiations when you're tired and vulnerable to the Willpower Gap, just one commitment to do what you chose when you were relaxed and full.

LOOKING FORWARD

If your Lines are wonky because of stress, overwhelm, lack of time, willpower depletion, or decision fatigue, a habit that I started a while back is picking the one most important thing that I have to get done for the next day. In his book *The ONE Thing*, Gary Keller writes about how helpful it can be to distill all of life's chaotic pulls on us down to one thing that needs to get done and focus on that. So often in this world of overwhelm and overbusyness, people fail to do the important thing because they're so focused on all the little things. I pick the one thing that I need to get done the next day, and I email it to a friend who does accountability with me. As I email her my one thing for the next day, I also check in and say how I did on my one thing for that day.

You might also have a routine where you look at a calendar for the next day so you don't miss any appointments. This is all to the greater good of reducing the emotional load that comes from stress and overwhelm. Emotionally self-regulating—or in common parlance, keeping your shit together—when it feels like you're behind, frazzled, or overwhelmed can knock your willpower down to zero in a matter of minutes. This is one of the reasons that parents of small children are especially vulnerable to the pull of sugar; just keeping calm in the face of crayon on the wall is all the brain can manage.

The stronger you can set up your day so you can move smoothly from commitment to commitment, the better. That might mean laying your gym or office clothes out, putting your office ID and keys by the door, and making your Bright Line meals the night before. Give your tomorrow the best shot it possibly can have to be a Bright Day.

LOOKING BACKWARD

As we look back over our day, we practice two cornerstones of Bright Line Living: accountability and gratitude.

In the realm of accountability, maybe you're responsible for bookending something from your day. Bookending is when we get support before and after a difficult event, and the check-ins are like bookends. Whether you made it through a gathering without breaking your Lines and now you post to your accountability partner or community, "Yes, I made it," or you are just recording that you succeeded today, "Yes, I had a Bright Line Day," that feeling helps reinforce that not only are you accomplishing this Bright Life one day at a time, but that it *matters*. Your person is waiting to hear from you. They care deeply that you are respecting your Lines for the good of everything about you that they love. Being able to end your day with this small moment of "Yeah! I did it. Go, me!" is so valuable. This pride is so hard-earned, and hopefully it will eventually completely replace any feelings of shame you may have been carrying for a long, long time.

The second set of behaviors involves gratitude, which is such a sweet and valuable way to look back on the day. There's so much research now showing that an attitude of gratitude really does train the mind to preferentially notice, remember, care about, internalize, and incorporate the good things that are happening in life. Way more is going on in life than we can absorb, and if we can train our minds to preferentially absorb the good things, we are the beneficiaries of that shift in perspective.

So once you get into bed but before you turn out the light, pick up your gratitude journal and reflect on the day a bit. If you've never kept a gratitude journal, I recommend you start with an exercise called "Three Good Things." The way it works is simple but incredibly powerful: each night, write down three things that went well that day and a bit about why they went well. It works because it changes your focus.

We are so quick to notice what goes wrong in our lives—an adaptive behavior that helped us survive before we secured our place at the top of the food chain. But today, dwelling on the negative can create a lot of unhappiness. Dr. Martin Seligman, professor of psychology at the University of Pennsylvania and author of *Flourish*, explains:

"People who are grateful tend to be happier, healthier and more fulfilled. Being grateful can help people cope with stress and can even have a beneficial effect on heart rate. In tests, people who tried it each night for just one week were happier and less depressed one month, three months and six months later."[25] The three things do not have to be big. They could be something as simple as: "I got off the bus three stops early and walked the rest of the way to the office to give myself time to reflect."

Then explore why it went well—why did giving yourself a few minutes alone before your workday bolster you? Perhaps because you carved out the time, you realize you are finally taking care of yourself. Or it might be that because you took actions yesterday to support your commitment, you fell asleep on time and had the extra minutes this morning to do something nice for yourself. That's what I mean by why—what explains how that good thing came to pass? What have you done, now or in the past, or what has someone else done, now or in the past, that resulted in that good thing manifesting in your life?

It's important to note that if you have a gratitude practice, you'll want to keep it fresh. Research shows that we adapt and become inured to anything that we do regularly. It becomes automatic. We use the force of automaticity to our advantage when we create powerful habits to eat healthy food at mealtime and say, "No, thank you," to excess food in between, but in this case, we don't want our gratitude practice to be automatic. We want it to be impactful.

That's why it's good to have several gratitude strategies in the bag and swap them out every now and then. Sometimes I write the alphabet A to Z and come up with one thing from each letter that I'm grateful for. My all-time favorite is pulling out a topic that's the thorn in my side at that moment—a work project, a disagreement with a family member or an employee, whatever it is that I'm churning over in my head—and writing a brainstorming gratitude list about it.

I've been married for over 20 years. Anyone who's been married a long time knows that every now and then your spouse gets on your last nerve. When that's happening, I write at the top of a page, "I am grateful for David," and then I write all the things that I'm grateful for about him, and, oh my goodness, at the end of that I am so changed. That's a good one.

If you're grumpy at your recovery, you could write, "I am grateful for my Bright Line journey because . . ." Honestly, you can use this tool to really good effect if you're feeling resentful about just about anything.

JOURNALING

Journaling is the act of supporting ourselves through writing. Research has shown significant health benefits to journaling.[26] And I want to share some science with you. First of all, it turns out that writing with a pen or a pencil is not the same as typing on a keyboard. Writing with a pen or a pencil activates different neural circuits, including more of the ones that we want to get in touch with to connect with our thoughts and feelings. And while I'm certainly among the crowd that can type way faster than I can write longhand, and it's sometimes really tempting to type, I write longhand on paper. A different part of my brain gets activated, spurring those reflections that help me get a sense of my deepest, truest thoughts and feelings. So if you're going to be journaling for the purpose of supporting yourself in reflection, it's important to do it longhand.

Another aspect of the science that I want to share is that you should journal differently if you're writing about a positive topic versus a negative one. If you are writing about something really challenging and you're trying to journal about it for the purpose of letting go of some of the negativity around it, it's important to write about it from different perspectives and different angles. This takes the challenging incident and diffuses the energy of it by creating alternative neural pathways around that original memory impulse.

But if you're writing about a positive experience, you don't want to dissipate the energy associated with it; you want to concentrate that energy. In which case, your writing should ideally be a pure reliving of the experience. Just calling to mind and then putting down on paper all of the details you can remember about the experience itself will strengthen and reinforce the positive neural pathways of the original memory impulse.

One approach to nighttime journaling is to encapsulate your day in a five-year journal. You will only have a handful of lines to fill in for each day, so it won't take long. And trust me: watching your life unfold day after day, year after year in this type of journal is an incredibly valuable and satisfying practice.

Having an evening reading can also be helpful. Currently, the one that I'm using and have been using for several years now is *A Year with Rumi: Daily Readings*, a translation by Coleman Barks that I'm finding so rich and poignant. I love to end my day reconnecting to the Great Mystery that is larger than myself. It minimizes the egocentrism of my struggles and reminds me that there is a larger force for me to lean into and trust. What better way to end the day?

THE NIGHTLY CHECKLIST SHEET

Bright Line Eating involves breaking a suite of long-standing habits (like snacking between meals) and replacing them with a more effectual set of new habits. The way we establish, monitor, and cement this new lifestyle is with our Nightly Checklist Sheet. It lists the behaviors—from writing our food down the night before to making our bed in the morning to writing our gratitude list—that are part and parcel of living Bright. Now as we rezoom, it's important to remember that this is a living, breathing, fluid document that should be customized and updated regularly. I typically change mine at least every three weeks.

Making changes in your Nightly Checklist Sheet ensures that it accurately reflects what you *truly* feel committed to and the areas you want to monitor. Having something on there that you wish you were doing in theory but aren't actually doing is hugely counterproductive. In my experience, people stop doing the Nightly Checklist Sheet because they use it the wrong way. It shouldn't reflect what you think you *should* be doing or what you *wish* you were doing; it should show what you *are* committed to doing, right now, as evidenced by your actions. If all you're doing is writing down your food the night before, not crossing your Bright Lines, and doing five minutes on a mindfulness app, then you have three things on your checklist. And that's totally fine. The minute your soul cries, "But wait! I want to be doing a gratitude list each night!" that should go on your Nightly Checklist Sheet as well. It will grow and change. Modify it often.

For years I've done a nightly checklist on paper, and when I've successfully completed something, I check the box. When I haven't done something, I circle the whole square where the check should have gone. At a glance, I can always tell if my week is staying on track. Research shows we will do the things we want to do more often if we are monitoring and seeing, in black and white, whether or not we have done them.[27] That's why it's worth considering an analog approach to this.

THE EVENING EXAMEN

Another evening option for tracking, measuring, and monitoring your Bright Line journey is something I call the evening examen. It comes from a spiritual tradition, but I don't mean it in a religious context. The woman who first told me she does this used to be a pastor, so it comes from that background. She said to me, "Susan, I feel like the Nightly Checklist doesn't serve me. There's something very rote and very detached about it, and I find that when I just check these boxes, I don't come fully online to consider my day deeply the way I would like to. So what I do is I have a set of open-ended questions on the order of, 'Was I my Authentic Self today?' And I write about it in long form." Note that she was retired and an extreme introvert, so her evening examen was one of her major forms of feedback and reflection to create a deep, rich, present, Bright journey. She loved spending time each night on that period of reflection.

It can be done in a journal, but I believe she did it on the computer and would drop in photographs or pictures and create an evening newsletter to herself, like a collage. And the artistic aspect of it fed her soul as well.

Now, there are going to be trade-offs here. I think the evening examen will likely serve introverts better than extroverts. And it takes longer, so it will serve people who have more space and time in their day, evening, and life than people who need the expedited solution.

But if you resonate with this idea and you find that the invitation to reflect at more length with more slowness and savoring sounds good to you, you could try coming up with a series of open-ended writing prompts.

CHECKING IN BY THE NUMBERS

My last suggestion for a modified Nightly Checklist came to my attention in a conversation I had with Dr. Marshall Goldsmith. He is the premier executive coach in the world for Fortune 500 company CEOs and the *New York Times* best-selling author of *What Got You Here Won't Get You There*, among other books. After only a few months of working with him, his clients up-level their performance dramatically, in ways that make them better people. He is focused on improving what matters. And he's a big one for tracking and monitoring.

I once had the pleasure of speaking with Marshall Goldsmith on the phone, and I asked him about his method for tracking. He keeps a list that's not too long, 5 to 10 categories or behaviors, tracking the hard things like "How much did I show up for my health today?" or "How much did I show up for my family today?" At the end of every night, he rates himself on a percentage basis from zero to 100 *out of what was possible that day.* Because every day is different. He might achieve 62 percent or 93 percent or 14 percent. Then he pays someone to call him every morning and hear his tracking from the night before.

The irony is that while so many of us are striving for perfection, he keeps one thing on his list that he almost never scores higher than 10 percent on, and that is "being present for each moment." On our phone call, Marshall told me, "I keep tracking that because it's what matters most to me. That I'm present for my life. On an exceptionally good day, I get ten percent. I reflect back on the day and realize that I've actually been online paying attention about ten percent of the time. On an average day, it's two or three percent." And we laughed together because I resonated with that feeling of being asleep at the wheel most of the time—even with meditation in the mix.

I, like Marshall, have sometimes found it helpful to put numbers to my day. I've done it by scoring my Nightly Checklist. For each box, instead of just ticking it off, I'll give each item a maximum possible score of 3 or maybe 5. Then I'll write the assessed number in the corner of the box and tally them all up at the bottom.

This makes it super easy to see how I'm doing. If I'm in the teens or low 20s out of 32 possible points, I'm floundering. If I'm consistently getting 28 or more points out of 32, I'm doing pretty well. By gamifying the Nightly Checklist, you can track the numbers at a glance. This is a *great* way to see if your sine curve is starting to dip. Solid numbers mean you're riding the peak, while low numbers mean you're sliding downhill and need to rally and get back on track. The numbers will tell you if you listen to them.

THE SEINFELD METHOD

The last tracking method I want to share is the Seinfeld method, which I got from James Clear's book *Atomic Habits*. The story goes like this: Jerry Seinfeld, arguably one of the most prolific comics of all time, would frequently be asked how he produces such consistently high-quality comedy in such volume. And his answer was that he uses a habit tracker to log when he writes jokes, and he strives to do it every day. His goal is to "never break the chain." Note that his goal isn't to write good jokes; it's to show up to the practice of writing at least one joke every day and never break the chain. A simple tracking system for this is a calendar where you put an "X" on the day when you do the desired action. This strategy of putting an X on a calendar out where you can see it and striving to "never break the chain" is incredibly effective.

I do my Nightly Checklist *and* I often have at least one calendar going that is tracking a particular behavior with the X game. And it doesn't have to be an X. A lot of people in Bright Line Eating love getting glittery, fancy, delightful stickers and using one for every successful day. It's remarkably reinforcing. Now, I also recommend having a way of noting if you didn't do it, beyond just leaving it blank. For example, when I miss, I put down a big heart. Because it's important to me to remember to have a sweet, tender place for my imperfections.

You can print a calendar, buy one, or create one of your own. It doesn't matter if it's August; buy a calendar and just start with August. The notion that you can't buy a calendar because it's not January is a perfectionist thought. Buy a calendar and just use the months you need.

TRACKING: BEYOND PERFECTIONISM

Learning to be comfortable with tracking our behavior without *judging* our behavior is where we learn to surf well above the Danger and Destruction Zone.

But how do we pierce that perfectionist bubble? The one that says, "I'm going to start tracking in a certain way, and from then on I'm going to execute it perfectly every single day"?

Success doesn't look like starting off perfect and staying perfect forever. What it looks like is you start off, and you rise up, and then you level off, and then you have small ebbs and flows from there. Ups and downs, and ups and downs, and *that doesn't mean that you're picking up the food on every downswing*. It does mean that things sometimes get a little wonky, whether it's your support or your actions or your habits. But because you're tracking and monitoring, you notice it sooner, and you go back on the upswing.

I want to show you a set of calendars from a particular three-month stint in my life. I used the Seinfeld method to track talking with one of my recovery support buddies and gave myself an X each day I talked live on the phone with someone. You'll see the first month I did great.

Sun	Mon	Tue	Wed	Thu	Fri	Sat
				1	2	3
4	5	6	7	8	9	10
11	12	13	14	15	16	17
18	19	20	21	22	23	24
25	26	27	28	29	30	

I had X after X after X after X after X after X and then I had this one heart day, and I was so bummed to break the chain of X's, but it really happened: I didn't talk with anyone that day. I had to swallow the disappointment and move on.

And then the next month, I had a lot more on my plate.

Sun	Mon	Tue	Wed	Thu	Fri	Sat
						1
2	3	4	5	6	7	8
9	10	11	12	13	14	15
16	17	18	19	20	21	22
23	24	25	26	27	28	29
30	31					

It was a holiday month, and a travel month, and a heavier workload month, and all of a sudden, I was really spotty with making those phone calls. There were X's and hearts, and X's and hearts in almost equal measure, and I kept tracking it, and I noticed, "Wow, okay." At that point, my inner voice said, *Okay, this is what it looks like right now.* I knew it was because I had a lot on my plate. But I checked in with myself: *Am I doing the best I can?* And the answer was yes. I was doing the best I could.

And then the third month dawned, and I was on the road, out of town, three different trips, back-to-back, spanning multiple continents, and I went for a long stretch with no phone calls to anyone.

Sun	Mon	Tue	Wed	Thu	Fri	Sat
		1 ♡	2 ✕	3 ✕	4 ✕	5 ✕
6 ✕	7 ♡	8 ♡	9 ♡	10 ♡	11 ♡	12 ♡
13 ♡	14 ♡	15 ♡	16 ♡	17 ♡	18 ♡	19 ♡
20 ♡	21 ✕	22 ✕	23 ✕	24 ✕	25 ✕	26 ✕
27 ✕	28 ✕	29 ✕	30 ✕	31 ✕		

I just went radio silent. And I got heart after heart after heart after heart. But then I was home from my trips, and I was able to say, "You know what? I really want to invest in finishing this month strong." So I went on the rezoom upswing and made phone calls every day to round out that month.

That's what real tracking looks like. Yours might look better, or different, especially if your life isn't as full as mine was during that stretch of time. But maybe not.

The gift of being able to let that calendar look the way it looked and decide at any point to hop back in the game and reinvest is something that I credit myself for. Because I know that tracking that behavior serves me, and I'm willing to let the truth be what it is. I fall off that behavior sometimes; it's okay. That's the ebb and flow of real tracking. It doesn't look perfect. It looks like data. And real data are messy.

But I cannot emphasize enough that it doesn't serve you to bury your head in the sand and not look at the information, because with real information there is always an opportunity to get back on track. The numbers being wonky or the X's not accruing on the calendar doesn't mean anything other than that you're not in a place where you're doing it right now, and it would be a good idea to watch for the next chance when you can. It doesn't mean that you're bad. It doesn't mean that you're wrong. It doesn't mean that it's all ruined. It probably means you need a little bit more support to ease the journey back in a way that best serves you, according to you.

You get to decide what things you track. Then let the numbers be real numbers. Not perfect numbers, *real* numbers.

And we will keep flying together.

IF YOU'RE JUST GETTING STARTED

If the idea of everything I have just laid out feels overwhelming, please start small. Let's just build a habit stack around brushing your teeth before bed. If that isn't even something you consistently do, then let's start there. Brush your teeth every night for two minutes for the sake of your future self and your dental bills.

Then stack one thing on that behavior. Maybe during those two minutes, you think through everything you are grateful for until your timer goes off, and that's it. That's *fine*. That is an absolutely wonderful place to start. When that begins to feel solid, add another habit to the stack—but don't pile on too many things if you feel like your foundation hasn't set yet. All of this is intended to support your food recovery—not capsize it.

TIMING

The timing of the nighttime routine is critical because you have to begin early enough to get a good night's sleep. As we are becoming increasingly aware, thanks to the research of so very many scientists, human beings have got to get enough sleep for the brain to operate optimally. And since the brain is the linchpin of everything we do, setting it up for success is paramount.

But for those of us who are in food recovery and wanting to prevent relapse, the sleep issue is even more critical, because research shows that people are driven to eat more when they're sleep-deprived. Researchers brought participants into a lab and had them sleep either four hours or nine hours a night, over five consecutive nights, and then let them loose to eat whatever they wanted on the fifth day. The participants who were sleep-deprived ate 300 calories more on average, while their energy expenditure stayed the same.[28]

Then the study put people in fMRI machines and showed that in a sleep-deprived state, the addictive centers of the brain are way more sensitive to food cues, especially calorie-dense foods made with sugar and flour. Essentially, the brain makes the body think that it's in a calorically deprived state and has an energy deficit and needs to eat when really it needs to sleep.

If you're planning your food out the night before and weighing and measuring everything you eat, you can eliminate much of that damage, but if you're breaking your Lines or returning to addictive eating, and you're not getting enough sleep, that might be something to look at.

In addition, when we don't get enough sleep, our cognitive functioning declines in ways that aren't immediately apparent to ourselves, similar to how we may think we're okay to drive after three drinks. As a matter of fact, our self-monitoring systems actually trick us into thinking we're performing even better than we are. The sleep-deprived person believes that they're functioning at a 9 when they're at a 4.

And finally, when we're sleep-deprived, our happiness level immediately suffers, and we're left feeling desperate and crispy and depressed and negative. This undermines our Bright Line journey because if we're not getting enough sleep on any kind of regular basis, we will experience our brain fighting against us. Tricking us into making exceptions or going into places or being around people where we know we will be tempted to break. The sleep-deprived brain eats more highly processed foods, and in larger quantities—all the things we're trying to avoid. If you want to follow your Bright Lines, an overwhelming amount of data suggests you'd do well to take the necessary steps to ensure your brain is on board, and that means getting enough sleep.

So how does this pertain to the timing of the nighttime routine? It means saying, "What time do I need to wake up in the morning to get my morning routine done and start my day on time?" That's your wake-up time. Then count backward. How much sleep do you need? Eight hours? A little more? A little less? Do the math. Now you know what time you need to go to bed. How long does your evening routine take? Maybe build a little cushion in there, and now you've got a shutdown time. Now you know exactly what time the technology and your day need to shut down, and when you need to start your nighttime routine.

For example, let's imagine you need to wake up at 6:00 A.M., and you need eight hours of sleep. Well, that means you need to be asleep by 10:00 P.M. Let's say it takes you 15 minutes to actually fall asleep, and your evening routine takes half an hour. Okay, that means at 9:15 you need to be shutting down your day.

For me, it's wise to build in more cushion. Maybe at my best, I can execute my evening routine in 45 minutes, but really, it's wise for me to give myself an hour, especially because I have to say goodnight to my kiddos. If one of my girls has lots of questions or wants to talk about something, I'm going to be needing some extra time.

After you've thought this all through once, give it a try and see how it goes. We're always scanning the instrument panel and adjusting our trajectory as we fly the plane. All the incoming data get put to good use.

THE KEY CONSIDERATION

As you are performing these simple little actions today that will help you with your program, yes, they will benefit you today. And give you relief. And assistance. And support. But ideally they do something way more than that. They set you up for a better tomorrow because down the road, when all these actions are automatic, that's when you'll really be on Easy Street. That's how you become someone who has left a crippling problem behind and is living completely transformed, shiny, and free.

As you begin to implement these actions, you may find that a part of yourself is incredibly self-judgmental. It thinks you're not doing it right or not doing enough, or it shames you for sitting on the couch, resting for 10 minutes instead of tackling one more to-do. This is your Inner Critic part. Most of us with food issues have vociferous Inner Critics, born of years of trying to bully ourselves into getting our eating under control or losing excess weight. As we get to know these parts of ourselves, it is important, as always, to stay compassionate. Being hypercritical is a strategy our Inner Critic developed to try to help us. It's time to give it a new one.

THE INNER CRITIC PART

If you are new to the idea of the Inner Critic, one way to get a sense of it is to ask yourself, "What don't I like about myself?" The stream of answers is what your Inner Critic has to say about you. If you can imagine these answers coming from just a part of yourself, you've found your Inner Critic. Now visualize what that part might look like. Is it a judge with a gavel? A harsh-looking teacher? Your mom? Your dad? How prevalent is your Inner Critic? How harsh is it in the way it talks to you? Does it call you stupid? Or an idiot? Or worse? Notice how painful it is to hear this from the Critic. What does it make you feel? Shame? Guilt? Anxiety?

As with all our other protective parts, the Internal Family Systems approach to working with Critics is to befriend them and coax them into changing jobs. They really do have a positive intent, even if their strategy is negative.

Remember how the Food Indulger gets activated when you are feeling stress or pain? When our Inner Critic is criticizing us, we become our own source of emotional pain. In this way, the Inner Critic becomes the prime driver of the Food Indulger. If you notice the Food Indulger popping up, check to see if the Inner Critic is active. Remember: "Don't shame; get curious."

The Inner Critic shows up for Bright Lifers in several common ways. If you have a perfectionist Critic, it may be shaming you for not doing Bright Line Eating well enough or not as well as others. You may even be getting wonderful results, but your Critic is telling you it's not good enough. A perfectionistic Critic drains all the color out of life by constantly comparing all that you do and are to some impossible ideal of perfection in order to avoid rejection.

It can also show up as the undermining voice that says, "You can't do this. You might as well quit." This is a very common issue for people starting on Bright Line Eating who are having struggles. This Critic is trying to keep you from feeling the pain of failure by getting you to quit. Or it might show up as a voice comparing you to others and then telling you that you are not a real Bright Lifer. I've had many clients tell me they don't reach out for a buddy because they have some deviation in their program (like using creamer in their coffee), so they think they don't belong in the BLE community. Remember: There are no Bright Line Eating police, and you are invited to make this program your own. It is just your Inner Critic telling you that you don't belong.

In their book *Self-Therapy for Your Inner Critic*, Jay Earley and Bonnie Weiss created a model that works with the Inner Critic and also with a part called the Criticized Child. It's important to get to know your Inner Critic (or Critics), but you also need to notice the part of you that believes the Critic's messages: the Criticized Child. We may think of the anxiety, guilt, or shame as our own, but it's really experienced by a Child part. If you get to know the Criticized Child *and* the Inner Critic, you can use Parts Work to transform them. In Appendix B, you can find tools to help you get to know your Inner Critic better.

If your head is full of negative, harsh voices, we want you to know it doesn't have to be that way. We've seen it over and over again: the self-esteem and self-compassion that are generated by a successful Bright Line Eating journey and sustained by frequent contact with people in our loving community can transform these negative inner voices into voices of support, encouragement, and care.

CHAPTER 7

SUPPORT

The last pillar of the Rezoom System is support. This doesn't mean *make sure your family is cheering you on*. It's not vague, it's not nebulous, and it's not a greeting card platitude or social media meme. Support is a step-by-step scaffolding that I will guide you to put in place to bolster you as you navigate your Bright Life. Support will help you smooth off those sharp edges, get back on the upswing fast, and build more and more cushion into your program so the ride starts to feel like a Cadillac on a freshly paved highway.

Many people in our community have found that, at some point, their relationship to food has interfered with making or preserving human connections, primarily because they avoided relationships out of shame—or because the people who loved them were calling them out on their behavior. Instead, they started to gravitate toward other addicts who enabled them. No other addiction is as easy to socially norm as food. Our whole culture is set up to support it.

While it's tempting to want to do the work of rezooming in isolation so you can present yourself back to the world at some imagined later date having "fixed" yourself and lost the weight, the fact is you need the support now. You may need to do a lot of repair work with people in your life to rebuild or repopulate your social circles with those who will support your Bright journey and the changes you're making. But you will heal faster and more sustainably if you foster and nurture your healthiest connections as part of your process and practice.

Another aim is to help you develop a cadre of support that you will lean on throughout a break and the subsequent rezoom. Personally, I have never felt the pull to isolate as strongly as when I've returned to addictive eating after a period of being Bright. I disappear. I want to hunker down, hide, and eat. Perhaps you can relate. But I've also experienced being able to reach out to one or two Bright buddies, people who have become dear friends, who I knew wouldn't judge me even in my deepest moments of pain and desperation with the food. It made all the difference. It helped me get back on track. I want you to have that.

HUMANS THRIVE IN COMMUNITY

Support is at the core of our Bright Line identity because humans are herd animals. Four thousand years ago, it was absolutely imperative to our survival that we stay with our herd. Also wired into our experience of life is a fear of doing anything that could ostracize us from our community. As such, we have a hard time sticking to our Bright Lines if the people around us who are near and dear to us are doing something different. And that's a big problem, because the reality—as you and I well know—is that out there in the world, our coworkers, our families, and our friends don't necessarily have the same issues with food, and they don't always understand the accommodations we need to keep ourselves healthy.

This is why we have to build a support community right here in Bright Line Eating. We have to, or we will continue to struggle. Because all the people out there who think that giving up sugar and flour is a little extreme, a little weird, a little different, or a little rigid (or perhaps a lot extreme, weird, different, and rigid) will chip away at our resolve. We can swim against that stream for a little bit. But long term, there's something deeply threatening about living in a way that everybody around us thinks is abnormal.

But here's the good news. You flip that over and it actually supports the opposite. Once we build a support community within Bright Line Eating, once we have people in our lives who follow the same Lines we do, who matter to us, whom we talk to on a regular basis, whom we care about, whose weddings we attend, and whose losses we mourn, we won't stop being Bright—because it's too threatening to our membership in *that* community of people who matter so much to us.

To build this community, the behaviors you engage in must consistently go beyond message boards. You have to get to know people for real, to the point where you care about them, they're calling on you in times of distress, you're calling on them in times of distress, and you wouldn't let two or three weeks go by without talking with them on the phone because you're invested in their life. This kind of deep support is the support that actually matters and moves the needle.

TWO SUPERPOWERS OF SUPPORT

In addition to fortifying our will to continue doing Bright Line Eating long term, social support has two superpowers that make it a critical component of the Rezoom Reframe.

First, it provides the most effective reset button possible in times of extreme stress. Human connection can ease that moment of tension when we feel really, really tempted to break our Lines. If we're in the middle of the battle between the Controller and the Indulger, there is nothing like a phone call or an actual connection with somebody Bright to get us out of that situation alive.

This is because support is the most effective replenisher of our willpower battery. We can be running on complete empty, make a phone call, get some love, hear somebody say, "Oh wow, sounds like you're really struggling," and be able to walk away from the temptation. In terms of the Rezoom Reframe, support is the key component in smoothing off the sharp edges. If we're tempted to say, "Screw it!" and dive into the food, or if we've just done something that our Food Controller thinks is questionable with our food and the panic is starting to rise, connecting with another person *right then* is by far the best way to get our inner kitten down from that tree.

But here's the thing. If we're not in the habit of talking with people in Bright Line Eating when things are humming along and everything's fine, we won't pick up the phone in that moment of stress. We just won't. That's why the habit of nurturing relationships, day in and day out, is key.

Support's second superpower is that it's the shortcut to developing self-compassion. Self-compassion is so important for us because when we break our Lines—or just come really close—it can activate the Inner Critic part that can start to beat us up, which generates a lot of shame. Our response to these negative feelings might be to hide, numb, and isolate yet more, and perhaps eat addictively as well, which of course agitates our Inner Critic further, creating more shame. And before we know it, we're in an out-of-control downward spiral.

Self-compassion short-circuits this process. In her book *Self-Compassion*, Dr. Kristin Neff describes the three components of self-compassion: talking kindly to ourselves, recognizing our shared humanity and universal struggles, and staying mindful in the moment so we can rally resources for ourselves. Sometimes this is hard to muster on our own, but the grounded presence of a supportive friend, whether in person or on the phone, can make all the difference. Their voice of compassion soothes us and helps us see that we're part of the human family, that everybody makes mistakes in one arena or another, and that we are not alone, not unique, and not flawed beyond repair. We're actually just garden-variety human beings. With their help, we can stay mindful and sort out the next right thing to do.

You know you're getting enough support if you're keeping your Lines Bright and developing automaticity, and if in the bar graph of your life, you feel like your support bar is higher than your stress bar, generally speaking. You'll feel like your program is *working*, and you'll feel deeply supported and connected on the journey. You're not reaching for the food to cope, and not reaching for the food isn't consuming every waking hour of your brain. Research shows that deep, meaningful human connections are the most critical factor in leading a life of flourishing and well-being.[29] Let's nurture that.

In Appendix A is a support inventory to help you assess where to put your focus.

THE SCIENCE OF HUMAN CONNECTION

Human connection is powerful, and science makes the case for increasing our support. There are three biological effects of rewarding human connection I want to share with you. The first involves our hormones, particularly oxytocin. First discovered in prairie voles, oxytocin is called the cuddle hormone or the love hormone. It's a neuropeptide, which means it's a hormone that also works as a neurotransmitter in the brain to affect social bonding and attachment. Oxytocin is notably released during breastfeeding so that we bond with our young. Those prairie voles? They mate for life.

Oxytocin also fluctuates during mundane daily activities, and not in a trivial way. These fluctuations impact our social decisions, business decisions, and self-care. A rise in oxytocin makes people 44 percent more likely to confide confidential information about themselves, and it also heightens our sensitivity to the cues that signal who is trustworthy.[30] We become more discerning. When we're in a social setting, our oxytocin tells us to trust, take a moment to share an extra hit of eye contact or a smile, and, as we're about to see, that can change us on a cellular level.

The second biological effect of human connection impacts the vagus nerve. That's the tenth cranial nerve, and it connects the brain to our organs, including our heart. You probably know that when something scary happens, your heart will race. The sympathetic nervous system tips you into what's called fight or flight: up go the adrenaline, the norepinephrine, and the cortisol; the lungs expand; the pupils dilate; and you are ready to go running really fast. The vagus nerve's job is to counteract that with its parasympathetic effects. The parasympathetic nervous system is the "calm and connect" nervous system, signaling us to relax, digest our food, lower our heart rate, conserve energy, and connect with others.

The vagus nerve is responsible for making sure we can experience a loving connection. It stimulates the facial muscles to enable eye contact and allow our face to show empathy. It also adjusts the muscles of our inner ear so we can track the other person's voice at a party. And it connects our gut, our heart, and our brain so that love flows right through our body.

But not all vagus nerve connections are equal; there's something called vagal tone. Vagal tone is the strength of the vagus nerve; it measures the degree to which our brain has a strong, calming connection to our heart and the rest of our organs.

Vagal tone has been studied for a long time, and it turns out to be a huge predictor of health. It increases the routine efficiency of the heart, fine-tunes the regulation of internal bodily processes, including glucose levels and inflammatory processes, and predicts the strength of our immune response. It also predicts how long we're likely to live.

What's exciting about all of this is that scientist Barbara Fredrickson has shown that vagal tone is not stationary and stable. It can actually be increased. The more love and connection we experience with people, the stronger our vagal tone becomes. The stronger our vagal tone, the greater our capacity for love and connection—it's a beautiful upward spiral.

Professor Fredrickson did a study showing that something as simple as reflecting back on our human connections at the end of the day can increase our vagal tone.[31] She had research participants take a moment each night to log the three longest social interactions of their day. Maybe one was with the checkout clerk at the grocery store. Maybe another was with their child or their spouse. Whatever the interactions were, the participants wrote them down and then considered them all together and rated on a scale of 1 to 7: *How true is it that during these social interactions I felt in tune with them and close to them?* That's it. This caused the participants' vagal tone to increase, and you could do the same in 30 seconds at the end of your day.

Because vagal tone is predictive of both overall health and longevity, having a simple way to improve it is tremendously valuable. It always helps to know what we're aiming for, and this way of looking at support and connection gives us a road map for opening our hearts, brightening our Lines, and living longer, healthier lives.

Steve Cole is a professor of medicine, psychiatry, and bio-behavioral sciences at the UCLA School of Medicine, and his research reveals the third way that human connection changes our biology. Professor Cole maps how our social environments influence our gene expression. People tend to think of our genes as being fixed, but scientists have been discovering that genes can actually be turned on and off. So just having a gene for a trait or disease (like obesity) doesn't guarantee that you're going to have that trait or develop that disease. If the gene lies dormant, it won't affect you. The opposite is also true. If you have a gene and then expose yourself to an environmental influence that hyper-accelerates it, not only will you be affected but you'll be extra affected. Thus, your genetic blueprint is just the merest skeleton, and your environment puts flesh on the bones.

Steve Cole and his colleagues studied 14 older adults over a period of four years.[32] Eight of them were people who consistently reported feeling socially connected—perhaps they played golf or bridge, saw their grandchildren, or volunteered, but however they achieved it, the point was that *they felt* deeply supported and connected. The other six people consistently reported feeling socially isolated. Again, this was subjective—the critical metric here is that they *felt* lonely. Then Cole's team scanned their whole genome, all 23,000 genes, and found about 200 genes that showed clear, systematic differences in gene expression between the connected people and the lonely people.

In the connected subjects, their genes for immune response became upregulated or extra active, meaning, for example, they produced more immunoglobulin G, our most common antibody. In the lonely subjects, the genes for the immune response were downregulated or significantly less active. But their genes for inflammation were on overdrive, and inflammation, as we know, is correlated with heart disease, rheumatoid arthritis, cancer, and the blockage of leptin, our most important satiety hormone.

These are not trivial findings, and they're not small effect sizes either. In fact, research over the last couple of decades has produced a shocking conclusion: feeling deeply supported and connected is actually more important to our health and longevity than the impact of *diet and exercise combined*. So, if you're thinking, *What's one thing I could do to stick to my Bright Lines and make my whole life better to boot?* then look around at where you can be in more connection with the beautiful people with whom you're traveling this journey. And then take it out into the world. Stop to chat with people in line. Smile at the crossing guard and say, "Good morning." These little connections are the substrate of your becoming a healthier person at the cellular level.

And happier too. Scientists Ed Diener and Martin Seligman did a study on extremely happy people, the most joyous among us.[33] And what did they all have in common? Every one of them, with zero exceptions? You guessed it. A proliferation of deep, meaningful, wonderful, fulfilling relationships.

WIDEN THE CIRCLE

As you consider the support you're getting, keep in mind that it doesn't have to be only people who are on a Bright journey themselves. Think about old friends, good friends. Think about family, maybe extended family. There are so many relationships that we let lapse because life gets busy. Are there people you'd like to be more in touch with? People you really adore, people who nurture you, people who get you, people who've known you for a long, long time? There is nothing in this world like an old friend. Are there any old friends or sweet family members whom you could reclaim right now by reaching out and making a phone call to them?

Other friends to consider are the precious people who know *how* to support you deeply. I have to say, some of my best supporters don't do Bright Line Eating. When we travel to entrepreneurial mastermind meetings, Ocean Robbins always asks me, "Is your food taken care of? Do you want to commit what you're going to eat to me? Can I support you in any way?" He doesn't have food issues himself, but he's a strong advocate for healthy eating, and he doesn't want to see me suffer, so he supports me in doing Bright Line Eating. He supports me in calling ahead wherever I'm going to be and finding someone who will bring me a Bright lunch or dinner. He says, "Can you get someone to help you with your food? You really thrive when your food is taken care of . . . it's good for you." The people who support us stand for our highest self, regardless.

I know that when you are beginning to rezoom, it may feel like you don't have a friend in the world. But that could not be further from the truth.

THE PHONE CALL EXPERIMENT

Phone calls, in my experience, are the magic. They are the number one most potent support. They create the cushion and raise the sine wave up so high above the Danger and Destruction Zone that we have a long way to go before we would ever break a Bright Line.

One of the strongest tenets of my recovery is this: connect before the crash. This means connecting with others on lazy Tuesday afternoons when all is well without a cloud on the horizon. I've learned that if you don't connect when everything is fine, you won't connect when it's not. When you make connection a habit, you have routines established for calling people. You know their rhythms. There's a deep familiarity there. That's the legwork that needs to be in place for you when you're triggered.

So I am going to give you a challenge in the form of an experiment. This image shows one week of the calendar you are going to use, and you can go to https://RezoomBook.com to print out the whole thing.

Phone Call Experiment

Date	/ /	/ /	/ /	/ /	/ /	/ /	/ /
📞	📞	📞	📞	📞	📞	📞	📞
Daily Rating 1-10							
Call Impact - +	▁▂▃▄▅	▁▂▃▄▅	▁▂▃▄▅	▁▂▃▄▅	▁▂▃▄▅	▁▂▃▄▅	▁▂▃▄▅

You're going to tack a printout or keep a digital copy of this calendar someplace where you will see it daily. You can leave it by the side of the bed. You could leave it on your desk or on your kitchen counter. Then your assignment is to talk on the phone *live* with someone supporting your journey every day for three weeks. The way the game works is that you get credit for the day if you talked on the phone with somebody. You do not have to be the person to dial the phone.

Now, ideally you will be talking to other people doing Bright Line Eating who are also trying to increase their support. Join our community, post, and find people to connect with. The reality is, people always love to talk with people who are walking the same journey they are. And if they're busy, they'll let it go to voice mail.

If you're someone who worries that you're bothering people, in Bright Line Eating we flip the script so that making phone calls is a service. You can wake up in the morning and say, "I'm going to be the person to help people out today. I'm going to dial the phone so they don't have to, and I'm going to have some conversations. We'll see who's around."

Next, I want you to collect some data. At the very top you'll put the date. Then ask yourself, "Did I make the call?" That's the box with the telephone. You can cross that off with an X or put a gold star on it.

If you miss a day, just like with our tracking calendar, I invite you to consider putting a heart over the day instead of leaving it blank because I want you to practice a certain form of loving acceptance. I expect that you might very well miss a day or maybe multiple days in this challenge, and that's okay. Just acknowledge it with love.

The next box down, the empty box, is for your day's rating, on a scale of 1 to 10; 10 is one of the best days of your life, 1 is the worst, and 5 is an average day. I want you to look at your day as a whole. Not how good the call was but your day as a whole. You want to look at subjective well-being: How well am I doing? How well am I feeling?

Then the next box tracks how the call contributed to your sense of well-being, if at all. If it didn't help your well-being at all, just make a mark right in the middle. Or if the call really gave your day a boost, make it a plus. If it was awful and bummed you out, you've got a minus.

Here are a couple of examples. Let's imagine you made a call and talked to somebody, and it went great. You had a great day, and all day you were feeling, *Wow. That call really buoyed me up.* You would recognize that the call had a strongly positive impact on your day. Let's say you rated your day an 8, and the call a strong plus.

Let's imagine, in contrast, that you didn't make a call. And you sweated about it all day in your head: *I should make a call. I should make a call.* It was a miserable day, which you rated a 3. And in this case, not making calls had a profoundly negative impact on your day. You're going to mark it as a strong minus.

Let's imagine you made a call and it felt like cocktail party chitchat without much impact to your day one way or the other. So you label it neutral.

Every day for three weeks, fill out those three boxes. Even if you don't make a call, you still need to rate the day. And then you rate the impact of not making a call.

As you're doing this, I want you to be writing down the names of the people you talked with; your goal is to build a circle of support. A circle of six people is a really sweet number, so that's what I want you to be aiming for.

And how do you know if they're your people? Because you like the thought of talking to them again. You really liked their feedback and perspective. It was comfortable and easy. Call those people again. Regularly. Start to get in the habit of calling them. Over time, you'll start to feel invested in their journey. Remember the precept: "Call before the crash." If you haven't been making phone calls all along, you won't make one when you need it.

The next step is to reflect on the number of phone calls that work for you and improve your program. What seems to be optimal for you? Is it a phone call a day? A conversation a day? Is it the case that those days when more than one conversation happens are a little better? Does it feel optimal to be doing a little bit more? I'm not talking about comfortable; I'm talking about optimal. It's totally normal if the phone calls feel uncomfortable.

On my Nightly Checklist Sheet, I have a line for how many recovery calls I make each day, and how many conversations I engage in. Somewhere in the range of three to five is optimal for me. I track connections using both the checklist and my calendar. But I'm an extrovert; introverts prefer fewer connections that go deeper.

Remember the biological, health, and cellular benefits of feeling supported and connected. Because needing to rezoom creates a strong motivation to effect change in your life, now is the time to make sure your conversations are happening in a way that is optimal for you. If you invest the energy to change the orientation of your support right now, while you're motivated, you will reap the rewards for the rest of your life. Plus, it's just a beautiful thing to stay connected with people on this journey.

MASTERMIND GROUPS AND BUDDIES

A Mastermind Group is a small group of about four people who come together on a weekly basis to support one another, hold one another accountable, and grow together in their journeys. I believe the mastermind group concept was first popularized in Napoleon Hill's 1937 book, *Think and Grow Rich*. Since then, mastermind groups have become very popular, particularly in the business world.

We've adopted this concept, and it has spread widely throughout Bright Line Eating. I formed my own personal Bright Line Eating Mastermind Group over six years ago, and we've been meeting ever since. We call ourselves the Magnificent Mavens Mastermind Group, and we meet once a week for two hours using a free teleconference line. We used to meet for 90 minutes, but for a couple of years we've been finding we need two full hours to have enough time for each person to share fully. Our meetings are very structured. Each of us gets an allotted amount of time to share, get support, and receive feedback. The mastermind call isn't a time to chitchat. Its value will be increased tenfold if you adopt a structure and stick to it.

For this example of a mastermind call structure, I'm going to stick to the original 90-minute format, as it's a good starting place. Of course, adjust as you need to, depending on your group's needs and the size of the group.

Mastermind Call Structure (90 minutes; 4 people)

1. Welcome each other. (4 minutes)

2. Facilitator asks who wants to go first, second, third, and fourth that day.* (1 minute)

3. Opening round: Facilitator asks each person to complete the following: (10 minutes)

    a) Right now, I'm feeling _____.

    b) My "win" for the past week was _____.

    c) Regarding my commitment from last week, I _____.

4. Facilitator sets a timer for 16 minutes, and the first person uses that time to share how they are feeling, discuss any struggles or challenges they're having, and get support from the other people in the group. A good practice is to share for 10

minutes and leave 6 minutes to get feedback and support. When the timer goes off, it's the next person's turn. (64 minutes)

5. Closing round: Facilitator asks each person to complete the following: (8 minutes)

   a) My "takeaway" from this week's call is
      _____.

   b) This week I commit to _____. (One person writes down these commitments in a safe place so they can be referenced the following week. People will forget.)

6. Scheduling. Make sure everyone can attend at the usual meeting time next week, find an alternative time if not, and pick a facilitator for the following week.* (3 minutes)

   *Alternative approach to the order and facilitation: rotate it so you already know the order and who will be facilitating each week. Whoever shared last the prior week moves up to first and everyone else shifts down one spot. The facilitator is whoever will be sharing last.

My Mavens enrich my life immeasurably, and we are incredibly committed to supporting each other on this beautiful and mysterious life journey. We never, ever meet if all four of us can't be there, and if our typical meeting time won't work, we go the extra mile to find an alternate time to meet. If you can drum up three other people who are as committed as you are, you will find yourself supported and buoyed every step of the way. It's priceless.

If you can't find three participants, get yourself just one person to support you—we call this "having a buddy." Your buddy is someone you can commit your plan to and call in an emergency. Many people in Bright Line Eating find that having a Mastermind Group or a buddy, or even two or three buddies, is the way to go.

FAITH

Another form of support that we don't often talk about is support from God, or the universe, or a higher power, or an unknowable essence: a certain bigger source of power, strength, comfort, and guidance that so many people tap into regularly.

You might already have a well-established religious practice with a set of beliefs and scriptures and a community that nourishes you, informs you, and is a part of your life and your Bright Line journey.

Or you might not be particularly religious, but spiritual, whether you believe in God or some higher power or divine mystery. Or maybe you simply have a sense that there's more than electrons whirling around. Something's going on here, beyond our pay grade. Or you might be atheist or agnostic.

If you're religious, I invite you to see where you're receiving support from your faith and to take a little inventory right now of the connections between your faith walk and your Bright Line journey. How do they inform each other? Does your conversation with God deepen because you're not fogged up anymore? Does this create an opportunity in the purer spaces to be connecting with God in your heart and mind? When you're tempted, are you asking God for help? When the temptation passes, are you remembering to say thank you? Do you thank God for all the blessings and miracles that are now apparent because you can see clearly?

I want to encourage you to bring your faith into your morning routine, evening routine, meditation, and spiritual reading. Really, every little bit of your Bright Line Eating journey can be sweetened if you bring your faith into it. And I charge you now with a lifetime of finding the ways to let the two inform, enrich, and inspire each other.

If you are spiritual but not religious, there are so many ways this Bright Line journey can expand your exploration of faith and belief to notions of miracle and coincidence, and to your lived sense of dancing with that mysterious energy. In particular, I think it boils down to coming to believe that some sort of energetic flow is shining love and light on you on a daily basis and is here to support you in being your Authentic Self and staying true to your Bright Lines. And if you're willing to believe that that's possible, a series of behaviors will flow from you that will form a relationship with this energy and divine unknowable essence.

It starts off by asking the powers that be for help: "Please take away these cravings. Help me get through this day Bright and shiny." Then if you can remember to say thank you afterward, you start to form a relationship. You will create a landscape for noticing when something is more than coincidence and the universe is conspiring to support you.

If you are atheist or agnostic, I invite you to consider the sense of an energy, a power that exists in the collective of people committing to their Bright Lines. We are all people who are walking arm in arm with you on this journey, and together we present such a force. The shared positive-supportive intention of these tens of thousands of people exists 24 hours a day, and with a post in an online support group or a text, you can access your share of that goodwill.

No matter your religious or spiritual orientation, or lack thereof, there is tremendous support available by orienting toward the unseen. Tap in.

PARTNERSHIP

Not long ago I was coaching a woman I'll call Bethany. Bethany was newly at Maintenance and was loving the transition to her Bright Body. But prior to her weight loss, she and her wife had a ritual of sitting on the porch at the end of the day, enjoying a glass of wine, and watching the sunset. She really wanted to go back to that beautiful, shared end-of-day ritual. So I asked her, "Where are you on the Susceptibility Scale?" She was a 9.

We talked more and discovered that the Caretaker part of her was advocating for her wife's perspective in her own mind and assuming that her wife would miss those shared evenings too much. What she came to realize was that her wife was in no way pressuring her. This was her own internally generated pressure. Her Authentic Self did not want to go back to drinking alcohol, and she wanted to keep her Lines Bright.

Once she reached that clarity, our coaching session pivoted to how she could allow space for grieving the loss of that evening ritual and the shared moments around alcohol, which was a big deal that shouldn't be glossed over. She decided to have an explicit conversation with her wife to craft a new ritual to create as much connectedness, togetherness, love, and symbolic symmetry as before. Most importantly, she would explicitly ask her wife for support. "This is a decision I've come to. This is what my Authentic Self is calling me to. I love you and I'm asking for your support." One definition of love is standing for the other person's highest good. Bethany knew her wife wouldn't hesitate to offer her exactly that form of love.

And yet partners and loved ones can have a hard time when we start doing Bright Line Eating and become devoted to it. It's a big change in their lives that they didn't sign up for, especially because food is such a bonding, shared social experience for many people. Having a partner opt out of a prior co-created, shared way of doing food is a very big deal. Learning to have intentional conversations about this shift can be really helpful.

Here I am going to provide a conversation script, loosely based on a framework I learned from Annie Hyman Pratt, the founder and CEO of Leading Edge Teams, who is a genius when it comes to having critically important but tricky, high-stakes conversations. When I started using her Failsafe Feedback Framework, I actually took notes, and I recommend that if you're going to attempt this with a partner or a loved one who's not so thrilled with your Bright Line Eating journey, you take notes and schedule the conversation. Let them know you have some notes that you've prepared for the conversation. I know it might feel a little embarrassing, but I promise it will be well received.

Start the conversation in a direct manner by saying what you want to talk about, and then share your positive intention for the conversation.

"I want to talk with you about my Bright Line Eating program so that we can get on the same page and both get what we want and need out of our relationship."

Neutrally reference something that just happened that gave you the idea that they weren't so happy with your program. Only mention the pure, objective facts about what happened, no interpretation.

"I noticed that the other night I was on my phone listening to a coaching call, and you said, 'Are you on another call?'"

Share what you were thinking or imagining without blame, judgment, criticism, or implying they were bad or wrong.

"The story I made up in my head was that you were unhappy with my Bright Line Eating program."

Say how you felt. Just be honest. Feelings are unassailable.

"I felt hurt. And I felt confused."

Acknowledge the impact on your partner.

"I've been thinking about what an impact it's been on you since I started Bright Line Eating and how you didn't sign up for this."

Describe the impact on your partner.

"We used to go out to eat and have long meals with wine and dessert. And we used to sleep in on Sunday mornings and have pancakes. I used to not have that many friends, so I wasn't on the phone that much."

Describe all the ways that you could imagine the impact on your partner.

"But I'm doing things differently now. And the story I have in my head is that it might really feel to you like I love you less or like I'm wanting to spend less time with you. And my

intention is for us to connect more, not less. And my request is that we co-create ways to connect in this new world."

Look them in the eye and explain to them the pain you were in before. They might not know how you used to struggle with food obsession, especially if you're high on the Susceptibility Scale and they're low.

"The truth is that I used to be in a lot of pain about my eating and my weight, pain that I wouldn't always share with you. Sometimes I would eat in secret and not let you see. I'd eat a normal dinner, but then I'd wait for you to go to bed so I could keep eating. This program is working for me. I know it's strict, but I'm finding a lot of freedom in the structure and it's helping me a lot. It's really, really important to me. And I'm asking you for your support."

Talk about new ways to co-create connectedness without food and think deliberately together about walks, movies, puzzles, board games, shows, and lovemaking.

"I want to be with you more than ever. I'm hoping we can return to those long walks we used to take. And puzzles—we haven't done a puzzle together in a long time. I also want to make love more; I'm feeling so much better in my body, and I want to share that with you. I'm curious whether any of that sounds good to you, and if you have ideas about how we can connect?"

Let them know that you genuinely want to hear them and find a solution that works for both of you. Share your hope.

"I'm feeling like a better version of myself, so I know our relationship can be better because I'm bringing a better 'me' to it. And I've said a lot. I want to listen now. I really want to hear your thoughts and find a way forward that works for both of us. I love you so much. You're so important to me. I want to hear you."

Experience shows that when they are approached in this way, our loved ones—whether they are partners, parents, children, or best friends—will almost always have a positive response. By showing such care for their experience in the relationship and affirming your commitment to the bond you share, you open the door for them to meet you halfway. Bring an attitude of humility, curiosity, and courage, and see what happens.

Over the years I've learned that while, yes, a recovering addict must prioritize recovery, that doesn't mean always putting every element of recovery, every day and always, above every other aspect of life. I've grown a lot in how I consider my husband's experience. I hope that I'm better at not assuming that my food recovery program always has to be, or gets to be, a trump card. In order for us to strike a balance, my acknowledging the impact of my program on him is key. And then he gets the empathy he deserves, and I get the support I need.

BROADENING OUR NOTIONS OF SUPPORT

The canonical exemplar of "support" in Bright Line Eating is talking directly with someone who does BLE and gaining a sense of shared connection and encouragement with them. In other words, person to person. But there are so many other avenues. We can also access tremendous support from the natural world, meaning trees and grass, views and mountain air, ocean waves and sand. Running on trails and digging our toes in the dirt. Closing our eyes and listening to the wind rustle in leaves. There are so many ways we can get nourished and filled up in nature. My favorite is to go for a walk or a hike with a good friend. Even in cities, there are parks and community gardens, and a majestic view of a downtown skyline is sure to elevate the heart. Nature feeds us powerfully, so much so that studies show we benefit not just from actual nature but also from looking at pictures of nature.[34]

You can also inhale deeply somewhere, no matter where you live. Think about what this means to you. Does it mean you need to plan a trip for a weekend, or perhaps a week, to somewhere really beautiful? Does it mean you need to take your lunch break, walk out behind the complex, and take your shoes off and stick your feet in the grass? Does it mean you drink your morning cup of tea a little closer to the window so you can look out and see the view? I invite you to take a moment and reflect on how you can be more supported by nature.

Last but not least, there is so much research on how our beloved furry and feathered pals bring healing, health, connection, and support into our lives. Do you have an animal or animals in your life that are providing you support? Can you take a moment in your day to register your love for them and your gratitude for the way they support you? I think it boils down to this sweet bumper sticker I saw once: "I'm just striving to be the person my dog thinks I am." Your animal always sees you as your Authentic Self. That support is real. Let it sink in.

SUPPORT FROM SELF

Yes, we can absolutely source support from deep within ourselves. And right off the bat, I want to distinguish this idea from isolation, because alone time, or support from self, is nourishing and peaceful and rejuvenating. Isolation is about hiding, about not connecting when connection would be helpful, which is a very different energy.

Introverts primarily refill their tank when they're alone. Extroverts primarily refill their tank when they're with other people. I use the word *primarily* because in reality, we're all ambiverts. We're all somewhere on the continuum, and no one is at any perfect extreme. We all need both. I learned this when I started the Bright Line Eating movement. Suddenly, I had employees and hundreds of people sending me messages all the time, which turned into thousands of people, all while I still had three kids and a husband, and a mom and dad, and in-laws, and on, and on, and on.

Eventually I found myself saying to my friends on the phone, "I feel like I need three days alone in a dark closet. That is what my soul is crying out for. Can I just be alone, by myself, for three days in a dark closet?" Turns out, you can do that. Not for three days, but you can check yourself into a float center and suspend yourself in a shallow pool of body-temperature water in pitch blackness with no sound, no light, no sensation, and you can just float there in salt water, supported, by yourself, as if you're in the womb, completely alone.

I now do that once a week for an hour and a half. I do that preferentially over a massage, over lunch with a friend, over any other activity because I need that alone time. A sensory deprivation pool is, for me, as pure as alone time gets.

And I'm an extreme extrovert.

There are two main kinds of alone time. One is unstructured, and the other is structured. Unstructured means an open block of time that you go into not knowing what you're going to do with it, but just that you're going to be alone. And then you fill it as you're moved to in the moment. Structured time is an appointment with yourself to do a specific thing. You could schedule yourself to go for a walk. Or see a movie. Or garden, or read, or knit. Or float. All of these activities, of course, could also be a part of unstructured time because they could just be what you end up feeling like doing.

What is the optimal amount of alone time for you? Do you have a sense of how much you need? Are you getting it? Are you getting enough support from yourself? And if you need more alone time than you're presently getting, is there a way you can advocate for yourself to get that time?

AUTOMATICITY AND SUPPORT

We can see our support through the lens of automaticity as well. I never saw this as starkly as when I stopped teaching at Monroe Community College because Bright Line Eating had grown so big that I had to hand back tenure and resign. For years I had been commuting to campus, and pulling out of the driveway was the cue for me to put in my Bluetooth headset and make support calls to people walking this recovery journey with me. Suddenly I lost that time in my day, including that powerful cue, and I found I was making a fraction of the phone calls I had made before. In that way, working from home was actually quite a loss for me.

It was important for me to think about re-creating automatic habits to bolster my support. I suspect it will be important for you too. Maybe our daily cue to connect is driving to work, maybe it's our daily dog walk, maybe it's that we sit in a particular chair and reach out to people at the same time each day. Maybe as we're winding down for bed, we log in to the Online Support Community and give people some love and encouragement. What has worked for you in the past? Can you build that into a ritual and repeat it until it becomes automatic? If you've never taken action around reaching out to give and receive support, I invite you to get curious about that.

Give the phone call experiment a try. Just try. That's one action you can take, and it's a potent one and perhaps all you'll need. But don't just make the daily phone call. Make it at a certain time of day, cued by the same, consistent behavior. Pick something that works for you—it doesn't matter if it's making the bed before breakfast or doing the dinner dishes—and repeat consistently for a stretch of time until it feels completely automatic. Your brain will take it from there.

The point, again, is that whatever actions you're choosing to build into your program, you do them the same way every day, meaning at the same time, in the same order, and triggered by the same cues. That's how you'll achieve automaticity, the beautiful state where your habits become part of your life and they support you with zero effort on your part.

I know all of this energy devoted to support sounds like a lot of work—but we have two choices in this arena of buttressing our food recovery: reduce stress or increase support. Beyond a certain point, I don't actually want you to work super hard to reduce your stress. I really don't. Because what would that even mean? For example, how would I significantly reduce my stress? Leave my fulfilling career and move away from family, friends, and neighbors? Drop the kids off at the orphanage?

There's no way around it: a rich, engaged life comes with stress. But on the bar graph of life, our support bar has to be higher than our stress bar, and developing the orientation of seeking and buttressing support is always the way to achieve that.

The main resistance to developing a good support system comes from the part of us called the Isolator. Many of us have well-developed Isolators who have been keeping us from much-needed support for a long time. But they've been trying to help. Understanding their perspective can be the key to opening the door to the support we need.

THE ISOLATOR PART

When we first introduced Parts Work to the Bright Line Eating community, we found that the same parts and the same issues would show up over and over again. When someone really had a problem keeping their Lines, we would ask them, "How is your support? Do you have a buddy? Do you have a Mastermind Group?" Almost universally they would say, "Oh no, I'm kind of a do-it-yourself person. I'm not really a joiner." "Oh no, I can't get into the online community; that's all too complicated." Invariably, the people who have the most trouble with BLE are the ones who have a part that isn't allowing them to reach out for support. We call that part the Isolator.

It's easy to see a part that is doing something. You probably connected with your Rebel, Indulger, or Inner Critic pretty easily. But it's harder to see a part that is *keeping you from doing something*, such as the Isolator. External support is needed for long-term success in Bright Line Eating. It's *not* optional. If some part of you bristles at this statement, *that* is your Isolator. You just felt it. Simply stated, your Isolator is the part of you that believes you'll be better off *not* connecting with other people.

Do you have a secret life? Many of us are familiar with secret eating. Our Isolator gets us alone, and the Indulger has free rein without having to deal with the judgments of others. When no one is looking and we don't have any accountability, it's very hard for an addict to be clean. Recovery communities are based on this truth.

Initially, the Isolator will try to keep you from reaching out. "No one wants to hear from you." "You don't have anything to offer." "You are too deep for these people." If you reach out anyway and don't get a response, your Isolator might say, "See? No one wants to connect with you." "You can do this yourself; it shows weakness to depend on others." Then when you do get a response, the message is, "Be careful what you say—you don't know if you can trust this person," or "Why would this person want to connect with you?" Notice if you have a voice like this in your head. That's your Isolator trying to keep you safely alone. By withdrawing, this part protects you from others' judgment, intrusion, and violation of your boundaries.

But it's important to recognize that not all Isolator parts keep us physically or geographically distant from others. Isolators can get especially tricky; notice if you have a part that seems extroverted but acts as a smoke screen to keep you mostly unknowable and distant. Perhaps your Isolator has you providing lots of support to others but keeps you from getting vulnerable and letting them support you in turn.

Inevitably someone in BLE will say, "Hey, I'm just an introvert. I do better all alone." But many introverts *also* have strong Isolators. If you are reading a book home alone at night and it feels great, it is healthy introversion. If you are binge-watching Netflix and feeling somewhat lonely, that's the Isolator. If you are doing Bright Line Eating and struggling and not reaching out for support, that's the Isolator. If you are walking in the woods alone feeling oneness with nature, it's introversion. If you have a lot of aloneness in your life and you are scared to reach out and make connections, that's the Isolator.

Just becoming aware of your Isolator is sometimes enough to shake off its trance. In Appendix B you'll be introduced to the different types of Isolators and invited to explore the ways you isolate yourself.

Coming out of isolation takes courage. But when someone who is struggling takes on the Isolator and gets the support they are missing, their program immediately starts to straighten out. You'll be surprised how easy it is to start to reach out and bring connection back into your life. What once seemed impossible will now feel natural.

CHAPTER 8

YOUR REZOOM

Many of us who struggle with our food and our weight have, at one time or another, surreptitiously studied someone in our life who seems to have it all together with their food. Someone who has a body that looks right-sized for their frame and genetics, who doesn't seem to think about their eating or worry about their food, and who never complains about their weight or their shape. Someone who eats one bite of dessert very slowly and then puts their utensil down with a look of deep satisfaction, saying that's all they needed. Such people, these days, are in a privileged minority: they are low on the Susceptibility Scale, *and* they don't struggle to maintain a healthy weight. Those of us, in contrast, who are of the ilk to have been drawn toward reading this book, have oftentimes looked at them with a mixture of curiosity and envy, trying to study what they do so we can attempt to mimic their eating.

Unfortunately, it just doesn't work for our brain.

However, while our neural physiology is different, there is something we can learn from those folks, even though we may never be able to get the one-bite-of-dessert experiment to work for us consistently. We can still look at the principles that govern these people's relationship with food because it provides a very useful framework.

The principles they embody are essential to our success as well, as essential as the acronym they form: AIR. *AIR* stands for automaticity, identity, rezoom. These are the requirements—for us, for them, for anyone—for having a healthy, stable relationship with food, eating, and weight. Those people whose brains don't have an addictive response to stimulating foods—they get all three for free; it just comes naturally to them. In contrast, we have to intentionally scaffold each of these principles into our life.

So-called "normal" eaters have tremendous automaticity around their eating. They have healthy rhythms and habits and generally eat foods that are in alignment with their values. Using my friend Nicki as an example, her life around food looks a lot like Bright Line Eating. In the winter she has oatmeal for breakfast, and in the summer she has muesli. Lunch is soup in the winter and salad in the summer. Dinner is whatever she wrote down when she figured out her meal plan the previous weekend. And she was eating like this long before she met me, not to control her eating (she's literally a 1 on the Susceptibility Scale) but to take food and dinner prep off her mental load as a busy working mom.

But when we eat whatever we want, whenever we want, we don't fall into automatic rhythms like Nicki's. So when we start our recovery, we have to construct our automaticity from the ground up—which, at first, is extremely uncomfortable and not what we're used to at all. But day after day, as we stick to the structure, the actions coalesce into little mini-habits, which then develop and strengthen into full-blown automaticity.

That automaticity really serves us on an identity level, which is the second factor of our acronym. People who are "normal" eaters have an identity around their eating. Whether it's "I'm a healthy eater," or "I eat for optimal performance," or, like Nicki, "I keep my food as simple and healthy as possible so I can have energy and time to focus on my life and my family," their identity around food is grounded as positive. And, according to Nicki, this also makes passing up calorie-dense, chemically laden, nutritionally vacuous food easy. She just thinks, *Oh, I would never eat that.* It goes against her sense of self.

We construct the identity of a Bright Lifer over time. It happens one day, one small action at a time. Those days, those actions, are the bricks that construct a glorious new castle-like sense of ourselves. This is what we do. This is how we handle our food. Our choices are motivated by a deep understanding of our addictive relationship with food. Abstaining from the foods that have driven us crazy in the past is what works for us. We develop a deep identity of someone who orients toward food in that way. The deeper the identity, the stronger our recovery.

Lastly, we come to the "R," which stands for rezoom. When it comes to rezooming, someone who has an unstimulating relationship with food might eat what we'd consider NMF ("not my food"). But they have a force of equilibrium that pushes them back to their comfortable midline. Nicki says she enjoys everything that's on offer at the holidays, or on a trip, but then in the days that follow she thinks, *Okay, enough of that*, and naturally gravitates back to her vegetables. For those of us who need to effortfully and intentionally enact this equilibrium—and perhaps can never maintain it if we introduce sugar or flour back into our lives at all—we have to learn to rezoom.

YOUR REZOOM ROAD MAP

In Chapter 5, I noted that your food might not be Bright at that very moment, and I encouraged you to rezoom. But I want to acknowledge that you may have read that section and simply continued reading without actually taking the actions to get back on track with your food. Rezooming can require an enormous effort, especially if you've been in the ditch for a long time.

In order to ward off the complacency that often sets in once we have months and years of consecutive Bright Lines, we have a saying around here: No matter how far down the road you are, you're always still two feet from the ditch. And in our online community, someone pointed out that the converse is also true: No matter how long you've been in the ditch, you're always still two feet from the road.

And although those two feet can be mentally very, very difficult to traverse because we have parts that drag their feet, akin to one of my young daughters who mightily resisted walking the couple of short steps to the sink to brush her teeth, in actual space it's not far at all. Like brushing teeth, the actions themselves aren't that hard either. And now, with the whole framework of the Rezoom System under your belt, you will likely find yourself enormously well equipped.

If you have a major rezoom to undertake, the first step is to take an inventory of your program—past and present. If you're embarking on a journey, you need to know where you're starting. Even a basic GPS won't chart a route unless it knows the address of your current location. You can take time in a few minutes to go to Appendix A and put pen to paper and answer some questions with absolute honesty. The inventories there will help you shine a light into the nooks and crannies, letting you see what's in the shadows.

If you've just had a break, the Permission to Be Human Action Plan, which I presented in *Bright Line Eating* and also in the Boot Camp, is a helpful post-break inventory to help you analyze what happened. I've used it many, many times, and I have included it in Appendix A as well. But if you've been off track for a while, the broader parts inventories in Appendix B are going to be most helpful. We don't want to let any jewels of wisdom go by uncollected. These breaks eventually turn into breakthroughs. You will start a successful rezoom by culling the lessons from everything you've done and experienced thus far. Remember the adage "If nothing changes, nothing changes." If you want it to be different this time, it means moving forward with full awareness of what you did in the past and what you're now going to do differently.

The next step is to set up accountability for yourself. Accountability really is the linchpin. Over the years of coaching people in Bright Line Eating, Everett and I have found that different people have different levels of what we now call accountability tolerance. For example, several years ago, I started something in Bright Lifers called the Gideon Games, named after Gideon, who accomplished incredible things with an unusually small and tight-knit band of soldiers. The Gideon Games are a 90-day contest where you join a team of 10 people, and your team competes to have the most aggregate Bright Days. Through his work coaching people in Bright Line Eating, Everett has found that a lot of people can't do the Gideon Games. Their parts won't let them. It feels too vulnerable to be that accountable.

As a result, Everett encourages people to build their accountability tolerance, to lean into whatever level of accountability their parts will tolerate right now and then gradually increase it. In my opinion, nothing is as powerful as committing your food live on the phone to another human being at the same time each day. And yet, that is going to be too blinding a light for some people. It's going to outstrip their current level of accountability tolerance.

If that feels like too much, just get whatever accountability your parts will tolerate at this moment, but keep in mind that accountability is the linchpin. Keep searching for a form that will work for you. Once you have your accountability lined up, the next step is to prepare to jump.

PREPARE TO JUMP

When you're in the ditch, the uncomfortable truth is that not every day is a day to get back on the path and rezoom; some days are just days to eat. That's not an excuse. It's an understanding that there are ebbs and flows in willingness, preparation, and mental fortitude, and that trying to jump when you're flat-footed is counterproductive. If you wait for the right moment, it will be vastly easier. So long as you're genuinely willing to be willing and the delay is just a pause to collect yourself, there's nothing wrong with giving yourself a moment to get ready to rezoom; it's actually wise.

Over the period when I was nearly constantly breaking and rezooming, I found that I had a part of myself, perhaps a Food Controller, that would watch for the moment when it could take over and get my food and my program back on track. It felt very much like when I was a kid and we would play Double Dutch jump rope. Can you picture that game? How the two jump ropes fly so incredibly fast, around and around? You can't just run into the ropes and start jumping. You have to stand outside and watch and intuit the flow of the ropes and your state of readiness. Similarly, I would line up my support and then I would wait and watch for the moment to jump back to the Bright side of the Lines.

As you prepare, engage in your own experience of watching the Double Dutch jump ropes by taking your inventories and lining up your accountability so when the moment arrives you can make the leap.

JUMP

Once you're ready to take the leap, once it's time to walk back up onto that path and rezoom, the basic actions you need to take are these:

1. Write down your food the night before.

2. Commit what you're going to eat, ideally to another human being.

3. The next day, eat only and exactly that.

Do these actions once. Then repeat them, one day at a time. You're rezooming.

THE DIAMOND VASE

In Chapter 4, I talked about Crystal Vase Recovery and Teddy Bear Recovery and how, when you reach the phase of automaticity where what was once the biggest struggle of your life now feels deceptively easy, what you have is a Crystal Vase. I said don't juggle it; it can shatter and then it never goes back quite the same way again.

In Sydney, Australia, I dropped that Crystal Vase and let it shatter into a zillion pieces. I did find it incredibly difficult to get it back. But I did get it back. And then, over a decade later, I ate again at that baby shower, which kicked off four years of having a really hard time stringing together a month of consecutive Bright Days without caving under the stress of my new life.

What I can say now—now that I have learned about my parts and how to stay curious about what they're wanting and needing, now that I've metabolized the experience of breaking my Bright Lines so many times that I truly couldn't even count the breaks and *learned a bit more with each break*, and now that I've stayed consecutively Bright for long enough that full peace has been restored—is that I don't think of myself as having a Crystal Vase anymore.

I feel like I have a Diamond Vase.

A Diamond Vase is similar to a Crystal Vase in that it manifests the tremendous value of a recovery program born of dedication, commitment, longevity, and focused, loving attention. And it's similar to a teddy bear in that it will never be left or forsaken. Having a Diamond Vase means that my program is working, that I am neutral around food and truly free from cravings. I'm in my Bright Body. I'm not obsessed with my food or my weight, and I'm not burning up willpower resisting temptation—because I'm not particularly tempted.

But unlike the Crystal Vase, the Diamond Vase is not susceptible to shattering. It's robust.

I do check the instrument panel several times a day. Scanning, always scanning. I write down my food the night before. I definitely meditate in the morning. And I make sure that I stay in close contact with my recovery friends.

It's easy. There's a flow. But unlike when I had a Crystal Vase, I'm not worried about breaking my Bright Lines. There's no white-knuckling going on over here. If I did break my Bright Lines, I would know how to get back on track. And I would be fascinated because that break would mean there was something to learn.

But I don't stand close to that ledge because I've been through a lot with my food and my food recovery and I don't ever want to find myself without my Diamond Vase. I don't want to put myself through that—especially the possibility of finding myself tortured by relentless food cravings again.

Could I get free again? Absolutely. Would the detour be worth it? Hell no.

They say that addiction is a progressive disease. It gets worse, never better. Well, I'm here to tell you that recovery is progressive too. Over any considerable period of time, with focus, effort, and a really good system to follow, recovery gets stronger and stronger and stronger. And eventually, you find you have a Diamond Vase.

Which means, in point of fact, that you have developed a Self-Led Program.

THE SELF-LED PROGRAM

The shattering of the Crystal Vase is something that happens when the Food Controller is running our program. After so many years of watching our food be a runaway train, the Food Controller loves Bright Line Eating and is so grateful to finally be getting the support it needs. But it also holds the fear that it will all fall apart.

A Food Controller–Led Program is perfectionistic and absolutist. Remember: our parts often think like children—in extreme or absolute terms. So the Food Controller doesn't see the distinction between making a reasonable substitution because, oops, the asparagus got slimy, or deciding to go out to dinner because your whole family is wanting to and plans have changed, versus simply eating something different for dinner because something else suddenly sounds yummier.

A Controller-Led Program is often a successful program from a weight-loss standpoint. But ultimately, it's a fear-based way to live.

Of course, we don't want an Indulger-Led Program either. What we're aiming for, and what creates the Diamond Vase, is a Self-Led Program. When our program is led by our Authentic Self, we trust ourselves to work our program because, when we do, we feel better on every level. And we really start to value ourselves and enjoy living in that calm, clear, connected, and curious place.

Our Authentic Self knows the difference between making a change to our plan because our Indulger is asking for something versus getting home late from the pediatrician and needing to throw a bag of vegetables in the microwave. Our Authentic Self knows that difference and stays calm in the face of life. This is where we're surfing.

Coming from an extremely rigid and Food Controller–Led 12-Step Program, I now encourage people to develop a Self-Led Program, where you trust yourself more and more and you're increasingly connected to your sense of strength in the universe and working to stay in alignment with your brightest and best good.

So you may have had a Controller-Led Program in the past where you were abstaining from certain foods but gripped by rigidity and fear. You may have had an Indulger-Led Program where you were eating off-plan all the time. With the Rezoom Reframe, you're being called to work a Self-Led Program, to tap into your Authentic Self and the tools that you've been given to live free— free of the food *and* free of the fear of returning to the food.

WEIGHT REGAIN

For the first seven years that I led the Bright Line Eating movement, I carefully avoided the subject of weight regain. Which is unlike me. I usually square my shoulders to hard subjects and address them head-on. Honestly, I didn't even notice that I *was* avoiding this subject because I spoke so often about my initial regain in Australia. But that was framed as the darkest hour before the dawn—the dawn of years of glorious, unbroken commitment to my four Bright Lines and losing all my excess weight for good. Problem solved.

I could talk about my one big weight regain in the past but I couldn't address it as a present-day reality in our community until the courage of JP Schiller. Here's the story of JP Schiller in a tweet: "With Bright Line Eating, JP lost 135 pounds in 11 months. And then he regained 150 pounds in 8 months."

Yikes.

He'd been on the road for a long time and then found himself in the ditch, seemingly helpless to get out. He had so many breaks and rezooms, it was dizzying, and compounded with the traumas of COVID, he had deep mental health struggles until it seemed like the Bright Life might no longer be available to him. But one day he turned the corner. And on that day, he reached out to share his epiphany with me. Here is the text he sent me:

I'm coming, more and more, to see the wisdom of the four Lines. All of my rezooms over the past 8 months have been: "No sugar or flour. You can eat whatever/whenever/howmuchever you want, as long as it's not sugar or flour."

I'm coming to see how deeply flawed that approach was, at least for me.

The meals and quantities Lines are important! They act as silencers to the food thoughts/chatter. My brain says, "Can I eat now? Is it time to eat? Can we eat?" And the meals Line says, "No, it's not mealtime. We don't eat right now." Likewise, my brain hounds me with, "Can we eat more? Are you sure this is enough? How about a little more?" And the quantities Line says, "No, this is the right amount. The amount our body needs. No more, no less."

Over time, our brain stops asking us silly questions like can-we-eat and how-about-more because of the meals and quantities Lines.

Without those two Lines, the food thoughts/chatter become so strong that eventually the sugar/flour Lines are abandoned with little resistance. And thus the merry-go-round of my break-rezoom-break-rezoom-break over the past 8 months.

Soon after he sent that text, JP proceeded to bless our Bright Lifers community with a series of essays, aptly named "Lessons from the Ditch." Here's what he wrote, along with a list of the topics. You can read the full posts at https://RezoomBook.com.

Back in October of last year, SPT and I did a vlog entitled "8 Lessons in 8 Months" in which I reflected on my time as a Crystal Vaser. Now, I want to reflect on my time in the ditch. I have learned new lessons and learned them the hard way. Now I want to share them with you.

#1—Sometimes you're not ready until you're ready.

#2—Up your support and strengthen your program.

#3—Be creative and try new things.

#4—Recover what worked well in the past.

#5—Do the inner work.

#6—Deepen your identity and stay close to the mothership.

#7—All four Bright Lines are important.

#8—Be kind to yourself.

#9—Don't give up and keep moving forward.

#10—Nothing is wasted in the economy of grace.

JP's willingness to go public about his weight regain snapped me out of my stupor and made me realize how important it is to shed light on the fact that, *yes*, in Bright Line Eating, too, people sometimes regain weight and *no*, that does not mean that everything is ruined and the program doesn't work. It's just another step on the journey of recovery. It's common knowledge that the average person tries to quit smoking multiple times before it sticks. Why would we expect this addiction to be a one-and-done march into the sunshine of perfection?

You might be wondering: What makes the difference? What's the sign, the hallmark that might tip you off that you're finally done regaining weight and this rezoom is going to last? Well, people are different, of course, and there's no one rule of thumb that will apply across the board, but I do notice that JP and I (from my time in Australia) both had the same deep feeling when we finally rezoomed for good. And that common feeling was *fatigue*. When you're beyond deeply, bone-heavy tired of being beaten up by the food, you're ready to surrender to working the plan, one day at a time. And in that state, a new level of honesty will open up so you can face, and address, whatever wasn't working in the past.

Each rezoom brings us one step closer to working a program that is strong enough to treat whatever level of food addiction we personally have in play. Once we're working *that* program, permanent freedom comes along for the ride.

MAKING IT LAST

Once you're solidly Bright again, the formula for long-term maintenance is simple. It's gratitude and service. Gratitude is two things. It's an action, like making a gratitude list, and it's a state of mind as well. In my old 12-Step meetings, the most successful members used to say, "Grateful hearts don't eat." You want to reach a point where gratitude is a state of being that hums in your heart at all times. Until you get there, take the actions of gratitude and watch your perspective, and your day, shift for the better.

The Stoics have a principle they call *amor fati*, which translates to "love of fate," or as Marcus Aurelius said, "To love only what happens, what was destined. No greater harmony." Someone once proposed a thought experiment on *amor fati*, and I've never forgotten it. It goes like this: Imagine you have unlimited power to create literally any reality you want. You have a genie in a bottle or a magic wand. Love this moment as if this, this moment right here, is what you would conjure up. Orient toward every moment that way, as if it were your perfect, self-chosen ideal.

Let that sink in for a second. It is incredibly profound, the gratitude for life as it is—all of it—the hard things, the boring things, the painful things.

From that place of deep, abiding gratitude, it's very natural to turn our attention to finding a way to be of service in our families and our communities. Right here in Bright Line Eating, can you be someone who takes someone's food commitment every day and supports them?

When my depression returned after not having been clinically depressed for 17 years, a friend of mine asked me about my sponsoring and I said, "Oh, I haven't been sponsoring in a few years. I started this Bright Line Eating thing and I started to feel like my whole life was now dedicated to service, serving thousands of people and trying to lead and serve all these employees, plus my kids, so with the time crunch, I gradually let go of my sponsees." And he said, "Yeah, well, you might want to consider sponsoring again." So I did. And my depression lifted.

And I did. For fun and for free, I started carving out 45 minutes in my morning to talk with three different food-addiction sponsees, 15 minutes apiece. And that was one of the things that resulted in me, as of the writing of this book, not going back to the food again.

We have an Online Support Community in Bright Line Eating, and taking time to go in there deliberately to offer support, to be of service, to orient toward not what I can get from life but what I can contribute is the orientation that makes a Bright Life truly possible.

Gratitude and service. They are the formula.

FINAL THOUGHTS

Food addiction is real, but it's not a binary construct. It's not an either/or proposition that we're either *food addicts* or *not food addicts*. Instead, there are gradations; it's a continuum—a notion we may have first encountered when we first saw the Susceptibility Scale. These gradations of severity highlight one critical fact: we each need to find our balance point with our recovery, where the program we're working is strong enough to treat the degree of addiction we have in play. When we find that balance point, our program feels congruent and full of ease.

We've made it our own. We're being restored to our Bright Body, or perhaps we've already transitioned to Maintenance and are living in our Bright Body. We're not experiencing cravings that disrupt our everyday life. Instead, the cravings have faded into mere occasional food thoughts that are easily shrugged off by turning our attention elsewhere or taking a swift action, like making a phone call or saying a quick prayer or mantra. We have habits and routines in place that support our recovery, habits that we soon discover are simply the foundation of healthy living. And finally, often the most rewarding and unexpected benefit is that we now belong to a community of people with whom we feel deeply connected and whose presence in our lives offsets the daily erosion of comments from unthinking friends, family, or coworkers.

For some of us, finding the place where we're working a program that's strong enough to put our food addiction into remission requires deep surrender and acceptance. Possibly, we're going to have to go through a fair bit of pain and grief to get there. We might really want to be able to experiment in certain ways with certain foods. Or we might have parts of us that balk at implementing certain aspects of the recovery prescription. We might wish that we didn't have this condition in the first place.

And what I want to say about that might surprise you.

The truth is that we can go down the path of nonacceptance as far as we want to.

It's our call.

There's an old Spanish proverb that has been quoted by many English and American writers, including Agatha Christie. It goes like this:

God says: Take what you want. And pay for it.

I think this applies brilliantly to our food journey. If we want to take a life of living in our Bright Body, free from food cravings and full of peace, joy, and purpose, we can take it. And we'll have to pay for it. It does mean surrendering certain foods. It does mean accepting a certain amount of discipline into our life. It does mean moving past our resistance and ponying up the effort to make friends within the community that supports us.

And we can go the other way too. If we want to make our exceptions and try our experiments, if we want to balk at the notion that food addiction is a problem for us, we can take that approach and also pay for it. For example, people say to me, "What if I don't think the term 'food addiction' serves me? I think that it's a label that becomes a self-fulfilling prophecy. I think I want to conceive of my state, my journey, in empowering language that doesn't pigeonhole me into a condition." To that I say, sure. As long as you're willing to pay the price, if in fact you have an actual condition that you're not willing to treat.

Take what you want and pay for it.

Ultimately, honestly accepting whatever degree of food addiction we have and surrendering to that framing and, yes, that label, can be incredibly empowering. Once you know what your condition is, you're motivated to treat it. Once you're aware, you become responsible. And because food addiction is the hardest, the treatment is a multipronged, multifaceted, interwoven system relating to our food, actions, and support.

For some of us, it takes a long time and a lot of pain to reach a point where we're willing to work a strong enough program to address the degree of food addiction we have on board. The good news is that with the tools that you now possess, you can explore the parts of you that might be feeling resistance to the fully expressed Bright Life. Those parts have valid concerns, based on their particular vantage point and their limited life experience, and if you get curious about what they are, you're likely to find things starting to shift. Which would be an amazing thing, because living Bright is so glorious that it's worth every bit of inner work it takes to get all of you on board.

And of course, this book can help. You may have breezed through it, but it was never intended to be a quick and breezy one-time read. Its true function is as a textbook. It's here for you, always. For your pen and your highlighter, your notes in the margins. You'll find, in time, that there are suggestions you weren't open to at first but now you are. Use this as your guidebook on this never-ending, ever-expanding, always improving journey where you just keep climbing and the vistas get increasingly spectacular.

Here's what I know. The more-than-adequate replacement for unhealthy addictive foods is the love we develop for the orientation toward continual improvement and ever-increasing growth. In Latin, the word for it is *Meliora*. Ever better. The Appendices come next, and they will introduce you to the treasure trove inside. And with your newfound understanding of the parts that are in play at the deepest level of your psyche, you will have a whole new approach to bring to bear when things get challenging on the path.

For someone who has struggled with their food and their weight, nothing is more glorious than living Bright. Meaning not just living in a Bright Body but in a Bright mind, a Bright conscience, and a Bright, peaceful heart. That is available to you in a way it never has been before, so join us on the path.

Rezoom and rejoice.

I love you. You've got this.

APPENDIX A

THE REZOOM SYSTEM

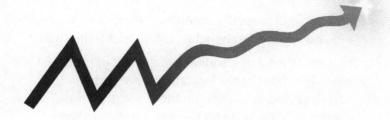

Food Inventory

Get out your journal and answer these questions. Or get together with a Bright Line buddy and take turns talking them through to allow you to slow down and really account for all the details. Be honest. And if you find your Inner Critic coming up, take some time to ask it to step aside until you can answer these questions without any part of yourself judging any other part.

To download these questions in a workbook format that you can print, go to: https://RezoomBook.com.

1. What BLE foods give you trouble sometimes (including condiments and beverages)? Do you keep these in your home?

2. What foods do you look forward to having? Would you say they light you up inordinately?

3. What ways of preparing foods can set you off? When, if ever, do you tend to have bites, licks, and tastes (BLTs)?

4. In terms of food preparation, what are your healthiest habits and what habits indicate you are closer to the ditch (e.g., batch cooking on the weekend versus picking something up on the way home from work)?

5. What's the ideal number of hours between meals for you? What happens when you don't follow that? What tends to interrupt or replace this ideal timetable? Is this within your control?

6. How often each week can you eat out and still be solidly in your Bright Line program?

7. Overall, what are your indicators around the foods you eat that let you know you're heading to wonky Lines? Describe the actions, as well as what you're thinking and feeling.

8. What is your pattern of eating when traveling? On what trips have you been solid in your Bright Lines, and when have you wobbled or broken the Bright Lines? What would you like to do differently next time you travel?

9. At what restaurants have you been able to get a Bright Line meal easily? At what restaurants is it more difficult to maintain your Bright Lines?

10. When you order a Bright Line meal out, do you tend to feel victorious or deprived?

11. When eating outside your home (e.g., visiting family, potluck dinners, celebrations, work lunches), what inner attitude or support system do you need to successfully navigate meals?

Line Breaking Inventory

---

1. When my Lines get wonky, wobbly, or crossed altogether, what tends to be the pattern?

2. Are there foods I need to let go of for now? If so, what are they? How do I feel about that?

3. When I'm at a restaurant, special occasion, or someone's house, do I ask for any accommodations in terms of substitutions or preparation? If not, why not?

4. What behaviors do I need to be especially careful around (e.g., eating out, entertaining, meal prep at end of a long day)?

5. Where do I need more support (e.g., time of day, levels of commitment and accountability, bookending, family pitching in)?

6. Is there an old idea preventing me from asking for more support? If so, what is it?

7. When do I tend to let up on the program and get complacent? How long do I typically coast before I break my Lines?

8. What inner resolve, decision, or commitment would help motivate me?

Support Inventory

What follows is a little inventory of your current support system so you can see, without any judgment, where you are now. Get out your journal and answer the following questions as honestly as you can. Or, to download these questions in a workbook format, go to https://RezoomBook.com.

OTHERS

1. What friends, groups, and communities help you stick to your Bright Lines?

2. Who makes you laugh and delights you?

3. Who really sees and validates you?

4. How might reaching out to these people more frequently enhance your life?

5. What old stories, ideas, or habits block you from connecting with these people more frequently?

UNIVERSE, NATURAL WORLD, HIGHER POWER

1. What practices, places, readings, or communities help you feel part of something bigger than yourself?

2. What settings fill you up with beauty or contentment?

3. What keeps you from making this kind of connection a priority?

SELF

1. How do you support yourself to be your best? To stick to your Lines?
2. What self-talk is most helpful to you?
3. What activities do you find deeply comforting?
4. What do you do or what do you tell yourself that blocks you from having more fun?
5. When do you feel most at home or at ease with yourself?
6. What movement supports your health? How often do you do it? What keeps you from taking that action?
7. How much downtime, unscheduled time, or time alone do you need each day? How much do you actually make time for?

What did you notice in your answers? Did anything jump out at you as an action you could take to strengthen your support? Again, there is no judgment, just a revealing of information and a chance to gather some data on yourself. But if there is an area that seems ripe for change, what action could you take today—today—to reach out?

Permission to Be Human Action Plan

Learning to live Bright is a process. There is no perfect straight line to success. It's a journey, and every journey has steep uphills, gentle downhills, and nice stretches of flat land. There are gorgeous vistas and horrible storms. You'll get blisters. You'll see sunrises. You'll go until you don't think you can take one more step . . . and then you'll go some more. Pretty soon you'll be a seasoned trekker.

One thing that can derail us is thinking that we must be perfect.

There is no perfect.

But there is progress.

This Permission to Be Human Action Plan is offered with love as a road map to follow in the event that you find yourself on the other side of the Bright Lines, and you want to get back on track.

Ask yourself these questions:

1. What was the situation? What happened?

2. What led up to it? How had I been feeling?

3. What sabotaging thoughts did I have right before I picked up the bite?

4. How do I feel now that I've crossed the Bright Lines?

5. Did I write down my food last night?

6. Have I been using my Nightly Checklist Sheet and other tools?

7. Did I take any actions to protect my Bright Lines before eating?

8. What could I do differently next time?

9. What have I learned?

10. What action can I commit to taking *right now* that will support me in my Bright Line Eating journey?

APPENDIX B

PARTS WORK

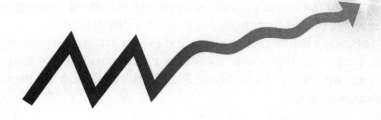

A BRIEF OVERVIEW OF PARTS WORK

To help us maintain our weight loss and our new ways of eating, it's necessary to recognize and address the parts of ourselves that have led us to our old ways of eating. Think about when you or someone you know says, "Part of me wants to be healthier, but another part of me just can't resist eating off-plan," or even more simply, "Part of me wants this, but part of me wants something else." In Parts Work, we recognize these disparate parts as significant and powerful segments of our psyche.

In Parts Work, we learn which parts are directing our thinking and behavior so we can recognize them when they're taking over. Once we recognize them and give them a title, it becomes easier to redirect these drives toward our goals, working *with* them rather than against them and turning our inner struggles into successes.

There are basic categories of parts, like the Rebel or the Indulger, but there are also more specific archetypes for each. This appendix provides an overview of the parts we covered at the end of each chapter and the underlying archetypes we use in food recovery for naming them and recognizing their subtle differences.

Following the overview are activities you can do to work with these parts and align them toward your eating and weight goals.

You can also find additional Parts Work resources at https://RezoomBook.com.

THE FOOD INDULGER PARTS

The Food Indulger parts are there to soothe us when we feel hurt, rejected, or stressed. They are perfect examples of the ways that food can be treated as a drug that covers up pain and emotion. While most people have one or more Indulger parts, these can be made more recognizable and predictable when we know the common forms of the Indulger that can show up. Consider the following Indulger archetypes and note which ones sound like what shows up when you eat off-plan.

The **Loving Parent** is a sweet part that likes to reward us when we're low on self-care. It often shows up when we're depleted of energy, after a hard day at work or caretaking for others. The treats it encourages us to have are replacing something else we probably need now or needed when we were children.

The **Impulsive Child** is impatient and wants immediate gratification. This self-soothing is common for children as well as adults. Similar to the Robot (Food Controller) part, the Impulsive Child eats without thinking. It sees it, grabs it, and eats it.

The **Seductive Rationalizer** makes up reasons to indulge and can be very convincing. It knows the perfect line of reasoning to get us to cave. "A little more won't matter." "Just this one time." "I'll do better tomorrow." "I'll eat less to counteract it." These can be extremely convincing reasons to indulge, and they rarely stop after "just this once."

The **Rebel Indulger** often shows up to balance controlling parts. The Rebel Indulger does not like to be told what to do. No one is going to control it. Like the Impulsive Child, it can be any age, and it developed to protect you by teaching you to look out for yourself.

The **Oblivionator**, also known as the **Binger**, wants to get lost, to dissociate, to lose consciousness and feeling. Bingeing is the activity, but oblivion is the goal. When we binge, we get lost in the pleasures of eating. We can lose time and especially lose track of how much we've eaten. If we're lost in the experience of eating, we are distracted from painful thoughts and emotions, and that is exactly this part's goal.

QUIZ: What kinds of Food Indulger parts do you have?

Mark the statements below that sound like what you do, say, or hear in your head when it comes to eating off-plan and indulging. The key at the bottom of the list will tell you which parts correspond with each statement. It is, of course, possible to have all the archetypes of Food Indulgers in your system of parts. For now, focus on recognizing which of these scenarios sound like your Indulger habits. Answer "True" or "False" to the following:

1. In the moment, I can come up with a dozen reasons why I deserve to eat outside my plan.
2. I refuse to eat the way somebody tells me.
3. I eat to feel better when I'm sad, upset, or hurting.
4. I feel like I cannot stop eating sometimes.
5. I tend to grab whatever food is nearby and eat it without thinking about what it is.
6. I make deals and bargain with myself about when to indulge and when to cut back on calories.
7. I like to spoil myself and reward myself with treats.
8. Bright Line Eating feels like someone is trying to control me.
9. When I binge, I feel like all my problems go away for a short while.
10. I'd rather lose myself in eating than deal with my stress.

KEY

If you answered "True" to any of the previous statements, it's likely you have the corresponding part listed below. There can be more overlap than just what's listed, so trust your own experience. You can use this quiz to better recognize, understand, and work with your Food Indulger parts.

1. Seductive Rationalizer
2. Rebel Indulger
3. Loving Parent
4. Impulsive Child or Oblivionator/Binger
5. Impulsive Child
6. Seductive Rationalizer
7. Loving Parent
8. Rebel Indulger
9. Oblivionator/Binger
10. Oblivionator/Binger

The Food Indulger Worksheet

These exercises will help you identify and work with your Food Indulger parts. Use these activities with the Indulger quiz to help understand and discern specific Food Indulger archetypes. For additional resources to help you with this work, visit https://RezoomBook.com. Get to know your Food Indulger:

1. Choose a familiar Food Indulger part. In your memory, go back to a time or specific moment when that part was active.

2. See if you can notice this part as a sensation in your body. If so, notice where it is and how it feels. Bring your awareness to this sensation.

3. Let an image form in your mind. What does this part look like? Where is it? Does it look like a person, a

cartoon, or an object? Does the part have any other sensory qualities, like a smell, a sensation, or a sound?

4. Now imagine moving that part out of your body and away, so that it's some distance from you (e.g., six feet away, other side of the room). Notice how you feel toward this part. See if you can lean into being curious and open to this part and what it can teach you.

5. Ask the part how it's trying to help you. Don't think or analyze; just listen in and see how it responds. Ask the part, "What are you afraid will happen if I don't allow you to help me in this way?" Note the answer the part gives you.

6. Ask the part how old it thinks you are. If it thinks you're younger than you are, update the part so it knows how old you are now. Thank this part for its efforts to help you. Tell the part that you can do the job of protecting yourself from now on.

7. If you are able, thank this part for its positive intentions. Know that you've begun to develop a relationship with it. Now do some journaling to describe what you've learned about this part. You may also want to draw an image of it, give it a name, and take any other steps that will make the part more real and personal to you.

MORE ACTIVITIES

1. **Swap indulgence for empowerment.** When you hear your Indulgers making excuses to eat off-plan, take note. The Food Indulgers want you to overeat or do other numbing activities. Instead, be mindful and centered. Swap out these indulgences for empowering alternatives, such as a brisk walk, a bubble bath, listening to music you love, an above-minimum amount of sleep each night, yoga, meditation,

and—just as important—connection with your support people. Accountability and human connection are empowering for many.

2. **Draw a timeline of your parts journey.** This can include your life prior to starting BLE, Internal Family Systems, or other Parts Work. Can you identify when in your life you've gained and lost considerable weight? Use colors, symbols, and drawings of your parts to show what has happened.

3. **Draw a picture of who you are and what your life is like when you've reached your goal weight.** What's the same? What's different? More importantly, what do you find that you expect to gain and lose other than the weight itself?

4. **Identify the strategies used by your Food Indulger parts.** They want to keep you heavy in order to protect you. Write about why they would do that and how they try to make you eat off-plan.

5. **Write a story about what happens in your life— internal and external, personal and public—if an Indulger part is healed and steps aside.** How do the other parts react? Does the system fall apart, or do the other parts work overtime? Or is there another outcome entirely?

THE FOOD CONTROLLER PARTS

A Food Controller part wants to exert control over our eating and the circumstances of our eating. It doesn't just want to control what we eat and how much; it also tries to control whom we eat with, who can see us eat, and where and when we eat. Our Food Controllers typically love the structure and rigor of Bright Line

Eating. Consider the following Controller archetypes and note which ones show up when you try to control your eating.

The **Permissive Parent** often doesn't seem to be able to control its Food Indulger very well. This type of Controller resorts to bargaining to try to keep the Indulger from doing more harm. Depending on the type of Food Indulger you have, this Controller may have little to no impact.

The **Perfectionist** is obsessed with doing everything right. Instead, perfectionism leaves us feeling "less-than" most of the time. If this part is super shaming when you don't perform perfectly, it might also be a Punisher.

The **Know-It-All** seems helpful at first, suggesting what you should and shouldn't do in your eating habits. The Know-It-All usually loves to tell *other* people how to eat while also directing the same expectations inward. Of course, having a Know-It-All part doesn't mean we've been successful in our food struggles!

The **Purger** shows up in bulimic activity, including laxative use, and is a part that may consider food to be shameful or even somehow poisonous. It must then expel already-consumed calories by any means necessary.

The **Punisher** is a harsh Food Controller part. This part generates shame, but shame is the fuel that drives so many of these parts, creating a chain of mutually triggering parts. For example, the Punisher's messages of scorn can easily trigger a Purger part. If you can convert food shame into curiosity and self-compassion, you'll interrupt this cycle.

The **Robot** part is one of the most subtle but effective Food Controllers. The Robot detaches from experiences such as eating and buying food and performs its function without thoughts and emotions. Dissociating from the act of eating is a form of control, which is the opposite of mindful decision-making.

QUIZ: What kinds of Food Controller parts do you have?

Mark the statements below that sound like what you do, say, or hear in your head when it comes to controlling your eating. The key at the bottom of the list will tell you which parts correspond with each statement. It is, of course, possible to have all the archetypes of Food Controllers in your system of parts. For now, focus on recognizing which of these scenarios sound like your Controller habits. Answer "True" or "False" to the following:

1. When I break my Bright Lines, I try to find a "less bad" food than the food I'm craving.

2. Sometimes I don't realize how much I've eaten until afterward. Sometimes I don't even remember what I ate.

3. I'm really hard on myself when I eat off-plan.

4. I enjoy telling others about insights and tricks for making dieting and healthy eating work better.

5. I do everything perfectly in my program.

6. I remind myself to drink a glass of water every couple of hours and remind myself of other daily practices for staying healthy.

7. I sometimes make myself vomit after I eat a lot, or I take laxatives, so I don't absorb as many calories.

8. I feel like I'm worthless after I eat too much or eat the wrong things.

9. I'm so ashamed of the way I eat.

10. I go through grocery shopping on autopilot. Sometimes I'm surprised by what's in the bags when I unpack them at home.

11. When my Indulger is active, I have little to no resistance to its cravings.

12. I feel so gross after eating that I make myself throw up to feel better.

KEY

If you answered "True" to any of the previous statements, it's likely you have the corresponding part listed below. There can be more overlap than just what's listed, so trust your own experience. You can use this quiz to better recognize, understand, and work with your Food Controller parts.

1. Permissive Parent
2. Robot
3. Perfectionist
4. Know-It-All
5. Perfectionist
6. Know-It-All

7. Purger
8. Punisher
9. Punisher
10. Robot
11. Permissive Parent
12. Purger

The Food Controller Worksheet

These exercises will help you identify and work with your Food Controller parts. Use these activities with the Controller quiz to help understand and discern specific Controller archetypes. For additional resources to help you with this work, visit https://RezoomBook.com. Get to know your Food Controller:

1. Choose a familiar Food Controller part. In your memory, go back to a time or specific moment when that part was active.

2. See if you can notice this part as a sensation in your body. If so, notice where it is and how it feels. Bring your awareness to this sensation.

3. Let an image form in your mind. What does this part look like? Where is it? Does it look like a person, a cartoon, or an object? Does the part have any other sensory qualities, like a smell, a sensation, or a sound?

4. Now imagine moving that part out of your body and away, so that it's some distance from you (e.g., six feet away, other side of the room). Notice how you feel toward this part. See if you can lean into being curious and open to this part and what it can teach you.

5. Ask the part how it's trying to help you. Don't think or analyze; just listen in and see how it responds. Ask the part, "What are you afraid will happen if I don't allow you to help me in this way?" Note the answer the part gives you.

6. Ask the part how old it thinks you are. If it thinks you're younger than you are, update the part so it knows how old you are now. Thank this part for its efforts to help you. Tell the part that you can do the job of protecting yourself from now on.

7. If you are able, thank this part for its positive intentions. Know that you've begun to develop a relationship with it. Now do some journaling to describe what you've learned about this part. You may also want to draw an image of it, give it a name, and take any other steps that will make the part more real and personal to you.

MORE ACTIVITIES

1. **Replace Controllers with curiosity.** When your Controller has stepped aside, you'll feel confident and curious about yourself and the world around you. Food Controllers lead you away from this confidence and comfort in your own skin. When you feel these parts taking over and attempting to blend, take some deep breaths. Do a grounding meditation. Then get curious about what's happening in your mind, your external life, and your body.

2. **Draw a timeline of your parts journey.** This can include your life prior to starting BLE, Internal Family Systems, or other Parts Work. Can you identify when in your life you've gained and lost considerable weight? Use colors, symbols, and drawings of your parts to show what has happened.

3. **Draw a picture of who you are and what your life is like when you've reached your goal weight.** What's the same? What's different? More importantly, what do you find that you expect to gain and lose other than the weight itself?

4. **Write a story about what happens in your life— internal and external, personal and public—if a Controller part is healed and steps aside.** How do the other parts react? Does the system fall apart, or do the other parts work overtime? Or is there another outcome entirely?

THE INDULGER/CONTROLLER POLARIZATION

The cause for the intense push-pull that so many of us feel as we try to lose weight comes from having one part that has spent years controlling our food and another part that has been pulling us toward the food. We call this the Indulger/Controller Polarization. This polarization often shows up as obsessive thinking when the two parts are battling it out in your head. Below are different types of "battles." Identify which ones sound familiar to you.

If you experience **Aftershock**, you're eating off-plan because the Indulger has the reins, but then as soon as you're done, the Controller comes in for that huge blast of punishing shame. Before and during eating, the Indulger may be the stronger part, but afterward the power tips to the Controller.

The **Passive Controller** scenario involves the Indulger knocking the Controller right out of the way. The likely Indulger in this scenario would be the Oblivionator/Binger. If you cannot find your Food Controller part(s), it's likely that this is the battle they're locked in.

In the **Plan vs. Impulse** dynamic, we have a Controller that likes to plan everything out: what we'll eat, when, with whom, and where. The Indulger is the spontaneous one, often a Seductive Rationalizer or Impulsive Child archetype, that eats capriciously and ignores or overrides the Controller's detailed food plan. The Controller part here is more active than in the Passive Controller relationship.

The **Good Cop vs. Bad Cop** relationship involves a strict Controller, such as the Perfectionist, and a very kind Indulger, such as the Loving Parent. Just as in the good cop/bad cop form of interrogation we so often see on television, both parts are working toward the same goal in different ways.

The **Abuse Cycle** involves a volatile or outright cruel Controller that fills our head with messages of viciousness, criticism, disappointment, and disgust. Once the Controller has reopened these wounds, the Indulger comes in to soothe the pain. If we have a really cruel Food Controller that bathes us with hate and abuse, the Indulger is going to jump in to soothe us in the best way it knows how—with food.

Public vs. Private involves a Controller that presents a public face to others. When alone, the Indulger comes out to binge or otherwise consume off-plan. It's common for the Controller to be running your eating when you're in a restaurant or at a party, but behind closed doors the Indulger takes over. This relationship between parts can involve lots of shame, especially when you're hiding the evidence of eating off-plan.

The **Breaking Point** relationship involves a Controller, often a Perfectionist, that is constantly telling you what and what not to do, and how and how not to do it. This Controller might be very harsh, but it could be more of a well-meaning busybody like the Know-It-All. Eventually, the Indulger finally loses its patience with the Controller and tells it to back off.

The **Seasonal Shift** refers to how, in a certain chapter of life or in a certain setting, the Controller will be in charge most of the time. Once this chapter or setting is complete, the Indulger takes over with a vengeance, or vice versa. This is common in snowbirds who might find that the Controller manages their food in one location, but their Indulger takes over in the other.

The **Transformers** tug-of-war occurs when we experience more than one Controller and more than one Indulger. The Controller may change from an encouraging coach to a screaming megaphone of shame. The Indulger may transform from a Loving Parent to an Impulsive Child. This transformation may happen from day to day or from moment to moment.

QUIZ: Which Indulger/Controller polarizations do you experience?

The following questions can help determine which of these common forms of Indulger/Controller conflict are present in your internal family system. This isn't a perfect test, but use it as a starting point for identifying the ways your parts work together and against one another. Mark "True" or "False" for each of the following:

1. Every time I indulge or eat or drink off-plan, I feel horrible. I feel like I'm the worst person ever.

2. When I binge, I feel disgusting. I feel so ashamed. Why can't I stop?

3. I feel trapped in a repeated cycle of overeating, punishing myself, and eating more to feel better.

4. I tend to binge, and no amount of criticism or planning stops it.

5. I tend to shut off my Controller's messages and choose the more pleasurable options of indulging.

6. Sometimes I'm great at planning my meals and sticking to plan. Other times I feel like I can't stick to it and want to be in the moment and spontaneous.

7. I get so overwhelmed trying to track and control my eating that I just give up.

8. I'll have a treat tonight, and then I'll skip a meal tomorrow.

9. I won't eat as much now so I can eat off-plan later.

10. In my head, I hear the same painful and cruel messages that I heard growing up. I eat off-plan to quiet that pain.

11. I'm great about monitoring my eating in spring and summer, when I want to slim down. I gain the weight again during the fall and winter holidays.

12. I can do whatever I want, as long as no one sees me do it.

13. I eat salads and other healthy foods in front of other people, but when I'm alone I get drive-thru and delivery.

14. I hide the evidence of my binge eating from friends and family.

15. I just get so tired of trying to do everything right! I need to be able to breathe without trying to be perfect!

16. I feel like my Controller was driving when I was younger, but now it seems like the Indulger is usually in charge.

17. My Indulger seems like a wild animal one day and a sweet, loving parent the next.

18. Sometimes my Controller is really kind and supportive, but sometimes it's downright cruel and severe.

KEY

If you answered "True" to any of the previous statements, it's likely you have the corresponding polarization listed below. There can be more overlap than just what's listed, so trust your own experience. You can use this quiz to better understand how your Indulger and Controller parts work in a system.

1. Aftersock
2. Aftershock
3. Abuse Cycle
4. Passive Controller
5. Passive Controller
6. Plan vs. Impulse
7. Breaking Point
8. Good Cop vs. Bad Cop
9. Good Cop vs. Bad Cop
10. Abuse Cycle

The Indulger/Controller Polarization Worksheet

These exercises will help you identify and work with your polarized parts. Use these activities with the Indulger/Controller Polarization quiz to help understand and discern specific ways these parts work together and against one another. For additional resources to help you with this work, visit https://RezoomBook.com. Get to know your Indulger/Controller Polarization:

1. Choose a familiar Indulger/Controller dynamic. In your memory, go back to a time or specific moment when these parts were struggling.

2. See if you can notice this struggle as a sensation in your body. If so, notice where it is and how it feels. Bring your awareness to this sensation.

3. Let an image form in your mind. When these parts clash, what does that look like? Where are they? Do they look like people, cartoons, or objects? Do they have any other sensory qualities, like a smell, a sensation, or a sound?

4. Now imagine moving those parts out of your body and away, so that they're some distance from you (e.g., six feet away, other side of the room). Notice how you feel toward them. See if you can lean into being curious and open to what they can teach you.

5. Ask the parts what they're trying to accomplish. Don't think or analyze; just listen in and see how they respond.

Ask them, "What are you afraid will happen if you don't do your jobs?" Note the answers they give you.

6. If you are able, thank these parts for their positive intentions. Know that you've begun to develop a relationship with them. Now do some journaling to describe what you've learned about this Indulger/Controller Polarization dynamic.

MORE ACTIVITIES

1. **Write a short story about the way your parts work together.** Are they colleagues in a workplace? Are they a family? Are they epic archenemies? You can also draw them to help make them feel more real and separate from you.

2. **Identify the strategies used by your parts.** They want to keep you the same as you are in order to protect you. Write about why they would do that and how they try to make you eat off-plan.

3. **Write a story about what happens in your life—internal and external, personal and public—when these Indulgers and Controllers are unblended and no longer fighting one another.** Does the system fall apart, or do the other parts work overtime? Can the formerly polarized parts work together to help you effectively? Or is there another outcome entirely?

THE CARETAKER PARTS

The Caretaker is so focused on caring for others that it avoids taking care of itself. This is a codependent way, rather than an interdependent way, of relating to others. The connections here may be quite superficial: a one-way process of caring that allows you to ignore your own needs. The Caretaker can look and feel like a loving mother, a caring son, a priest or religious leader, or a nurse. Many of those in service careers (such as teaching, nursing, military, clergy, hospitality) have a strong Caretaker part.

The **24-Hour Nurse** finds ways to interact with others frequently without actually letting them in. This Caretaker is constantly there for others: guiding them, comforting them, keeping them safe. This may seem like a virtuous way to live, but it is also a way to avoid accepting our own vulnerability. The 24-Hour Nurse avoids asking for help, as well as helping itself.

The **Pushover** is a Caretaker part that has difficulty saying no. Whereas the 24-Hour Nurse is mostly concerned with those who truly need assistance, the Pushover is afraid of hurting others' feelings or being rejected.

The **Martyr** is very similar to the 24-Hour Nurse but with a different attitude. While the 24-Hour Nurse seeks to prove its worth and avoid self-reflection by helping others constantly, the Martyr gives until it's exhausted and then pushes others away for not being more grateful. This resentment is yet another strategy to avoid personal growth and responsibility.

The **Pleaser** wants to avoid others' disappointment in it. If your primary goal in your interactions is for the other to be happy and satisfied, regardless of your own satisfaction, it's a sign that you have this part. The Pleaser is a master at conflict avoidance—it will never share its true feelings if it would create sadness or disappointment. The Pleaser is often secretly upset or resentful since it never gets its way, similar to the Martyr above.

The **Hero** activates to focus on helping others during crises at the expense of itself. This can cause resentment toward those who don't want to be helped or don't show appreciation. A Hero part also distracts from self-care and realistic, clear thinking.

The **Peacemaker** wants to avoid conflict. Conflict is uncomfortable for the Peacemaker, whether it is involved in the conflict directly or is just nearby. The Peacemaker will do whatever is necessary to keep the peace, whether that means surrendering, interfering, distracting, or apologizing.

QUIZ: What kinds of Caretaker parts do you have?

Mark the statements below that sound like what you do, say, or hear in your head when it comes to taking care of others. The key at the bottom of the list will tell you which parts correspond with each statement. It is, of course, possible to have all the archetypes of Caretakers in your system of parts. For now, focus on recognizing which of these scenarios sound like your Caretaker habits. Answer "True" or "False" to the following:

1. I don't have time right now to ask for help.

2. Everyone disappoints me eventually.

3. I can't go out or have fun with others. I have to take care of someone else.

4. It's important to take care of others. It feels like I'm doing the right thing.

5. People are so selfish. No one appreciates what I do.

6. I give in after saying no to people.

7. I don't want anyone to get their feelings hurt, even if I have to take the loss.

8. Why don't people let me help them?

9. I will avoid confrontation even when I know I'm reasonable or right.

10. I'm quick to rescue friends, family, or partners/lovers.

11. Disabled people get offended when I try to help them.

12. I wish I had more time and energy for myself when I'm done helping others.

13. I don't want to be a burden on others.

14. My needs aren't that important.

15. It's selfish to ask others for help with this.

16. I get anxious thinking about others being upset with me.

17. I usually keep my opinions to myself to avoid conflict.

KEY

If you answered "True" to any of the previous statements, it's likely you have the corresponding part listed below. There can be more overlap than just what's listed, so trust your own experience. You can use this quiz to better recognize, understand, and work with your Caretaker parts.

1. 24-Hour Nurse
2. Martyr
3. 24-Hour Nurse
4. 24-Hour Nurse
5. Martyr
6. Pushover
7. Peacemaker or Pleaser
8. Hero
9. Peacemaker
10. Hero
11. Hero
12. 24-Hour Nurse
13. Pushover
14. Pushover
15. 24-Hour Nurse
16. Pleaser
17. Pleaser

The Caretaker Worksheet

These exercises will help you identify and work with your Caretaker parts. Use these activities with the Caretaker quiz to help understand and discern specific Caretaker archetypes. For additional resources to help you with this work, visit https://RezoomBook.com. Get to know your Caretaker:

1. Choose a familiar Caretaker part. In your memory, go back to a time or specific moment when that part was active.

2. See if you can notice this part as a sensation in your body. If so, notice where it is and how it feels. Bring your awareness to this sensation.

3. Let an image form in your mind. What does this part look like? Where is it? Does it look like a person, a cartoon, or an object? Does the part have any other sensory qualities, like a smell, a sensation, or a sound?

4. Now imagine moving that part out of your body and away, so that it's some distance from you (e.g., six feet away, other side of the room). Notice how you feel toward this part. See if you can lean into being curious and open to this part and what it can teach you.

5. Ask the part how it's trying to help you. Don't think or analyze; just listen in and see how it responds. Ask the part, "What are you afraid will happen if you don't help me in this way?" Note the answer the part gives you.

6. Ask the part how old it thinks you are. If it thinks you're younger than you are, update the part so it knows how old you are now. Thank this part for its efforts to help you. Tell the part that you can do the job of protecting yourself from now on.

7. If you are able, thank this part for its positive intentions. Know that you've begun to develop a relationship with it. Now do some journaling to describe what you've learned about this part. You may also want to draw an image of it, give it a name, and take any other steps that will make the part more real and personal to you.

MORE ACTIVITIES

1. **Identify your own needs.** At some point in your early life, you learned that others' needs were more important than your own. Make a list of what you need—emotionally, mentally, physically, materially, and spiritually. Then, keeping emotional safety in mind, write about a time in childhood or adolescence when you needed support and connection but your needs were denied. What did you do? What beliefs did you form?

2. **Make a connection map of all the people in your support network.** If the support only goes in one direction (e.g., you're not giving any support back to the other party, or the other party isn't supporting you), make those lines in a particular color or pattern (such as a dotted line). Go ahead and connect these individuals to each other as well if there are support connections among them. What do you notice about this map? How connected and supported are you compared to the others on this web? With whom do you have a truly mutual support relationship?

3. **Identify the strategies used by your Caretaker parts.** What are all the ways these parts work to protect you and keep you isolated? When did the Caretaker parts really start to show up in your life?

4. **Write a story about what happens in your life— internal and external, personal and public—if a Caretaker part is healed and kept unblended.** How

do the other parts react? Does the system fall apart, or do the other parts work overtime? Or is there another outcome entirely? Who would you be if you no longer believed you need to take care of others at the expense of your own needs?

THE REBEL PARTS

Rebel parts resist, saying things like, "You can't make me do that," and "You're not the boss of me." Unlike healthy boundaries, Rebel parts keep us stuck in the same patterns of thinking and acting.

The **Angry Teenager** is a part that sticks around after adolescence. While trying to assert independence and self-sufficiency, the Angry Teenager will reject mentors, guidance, and authority figures. This Rebel archetype often feels that anger in response to recovery. You can find out whom or what it's rebelling against if you separate yourself from this part and update it about your current age. Let it know you're truly in charge.

The **Underachiever** never puts 100 percent commitment into anything. It tells us that a goal is too much work and that we can't possibly do it. The Underachiever part can be healed through external support, especially in the BLE community.

The **Questioner** part, unlike the others, comes across as analytical and thoughtful. This part wants to understand what's being asked and needs to agree with the goal in order to accept and do it. External support can keep it from second-guessing everything.

The **Dominant** part is immovable, even more than the Angry Teenager. It will not be controlled by anyone, ever. This part has some serious emotional and psychological wounds and weak spots that it is hiding and protecting. To appease this part, you can make BLE into your own personalized program to work *with* the Dominant part.

The **Butterfly** seems flighty, but it's quite sophisticated. This part keeps us from focusing and completing our goals by distracting us. These distractions prevent follow-through and lead to us breaking rules "accidentally" by losing focus. When you feel like you cannot concentrate on BLE, get curious about this part and see if you can get it to step aside. Accountability and external support will help.

QUIZ: What kinds of Rebel parts do you have?

Which of these parts show up for you when you're trying to trust advice, a plan, or a program? Mark the statements below that sound like what you do, say, or hear in your head when it comes to feeling controlled or bossed around. The key at the bottom of the list will tell you which parts correspond with each statement. It is, of course, possible to have all the archetypes of Rebels in your system of parts. For now, focus on recognizing which of these scenarios sound like your Rebel habits. Answer "True" or "False" to the following:

1. I don't want to, so I won't.
2. I've done enough. I'm through here.
3. It's not that important.
4. This is too much work.
5. Sometimes I feel like I rebel just for the sake of rebelling.
6. I often don't pay attention, and I eat off-plan accidentally.

7. I want to complete this, but I can't seem to make that happen.

8. When I try to focus and plan, my mind wanders off completely.

9. But *why* is this necessary?

10. I need to do more research before I agree.

11. I don't know if I trust this program.

12. I hate being told what to do.

13. I said no, and I won't repeat myself.

14. I will not be swayed or convinced.

15. I always win.

16. Leave me alone. I know what I'm doing.

KEY

If you answered "True" to any of the previous statements, it's likely you have the corresponding part listed below. There can be more overlap than just what's listed, so trust your own experience. You can use this quiz to better recognize, understand, and work with your Rebel parts.

1. Angry Teenager or Dominant
2. Underachiever
3. Underachiever
4. Underachiever
5. Angry Teenager
6. Butterfly
7. Butterfly
8. Butterfly

9. Questioner
10. Questioner
11. Questioner
12. Dominant
13. Dominant
14. Dominant
15. Dominant
16. Angry Teenager

The Rebel Worksheet

These exercises will help you identify and work with your Rebel parts. Use these activities with the Rebel quiz to help understand and discern specific Rebel archetypes. For additional resources to help you with this work, visit https://RezoomBook.com.

Get to know your Rebel:

1. Choose a familiar Rebel part. In your memory, go back to a time or specific moment when that part was active.

2. See if you can notice this part as a sensation in your body. If so, notice where it is and how it feels. Bring your awareness to this sensation.

3. Let an image form in your mind. What does this part look like? Where is it? Does it look like a person, a cartoon, or an object? Does the part have any other sensory qualities, like a smell, a sensation, or a sound?

4. Now imagine moving that part out of your body and away, so that it's some distance from you (e.g., six feet away, other side of the room). Notice how you feel toward this part. See if you can lean into being curious and open to this part and what it can teach you.

5. Ask the part how it's trying to help you. Don't think or analyze; just listen in and see how it responds. Ask the part, "What are you afraid will happen if you don't help me in this way?" Note the answer the part gives you.

6. Ask the part how old it thinks you are. If it thinks you're younger than you are, update the part so it knows how old you are now. Thank this part for its efforts to help you. Tell the part that you can do the job of protecting yourself from now on.

7. If you are able, thank this part for its positive intentions. Know that you've begun to develop a relationship with it. Now do some journaling to describe what you've learned about this part. You may also want to draw an image of it, give it a name, and take any other steps that will make the part more real and personal to you.

MORE ACTIVITIES

1. **Redefine rebellion.** What if your Rebel parts could do their job in a way that helps you in BLE? Teach your Rebels to reject the Standard American Diet rather than rejecting BLE. Work with these parts and make BLE your own individualized program.

2. **Modify the program.** What feels fun, good, and right about BLE? Check in with yourself by asking yourself the following questions about making changes to your program:

   A. Does this bring me peace or disrupt my peace?

   B. Is this healthy?

   C. Does this mess with my weight?

   D. Is this escalating?

3. **Practice ODAAT: one day at a time.** Remind yourself and your parts that you don't have to do this perfectly. Instead of focusing on how long this journey will be or how intense it may become, focus on just sticking to your program today. This makes maintaining BLE feel much more possible. Just keep going. You can think about tomorrow when tomorrow comes.

4. **Identify the strategies used by your Rebel parts.** They want to keep you the same in order to protect you.

Write about why they would do that and how they try to make you resist your eating plan.

5. **Write a story about what happens in your life—internal and external, personal and public—if a Rebel part is healed and kept distinct from your thinking.** How do the other parts react? Does the system fall apart, or do the other parts work overtime? Or is there another outcome entirely?

THE INNER CRITIC PARTS

Our Inner Critic work borrows from Jay Earley and Bonnie Weiss's brilliant book *Freedom from Your Inner Critic: A Self-Therapy Approach* (included with permission).

Inner Critics are parts that try to protect us by shaping us. They restrain us from certain actions and emotions to keep us safe. This was learned in childhood, often from an abusive and/or neglectful parent, caregiver, sibling, or peer.

The **Perfectionist** is an overachiever part that often thinks that if we look and act perfect, everything will finally go right. This part tells you, "Perfect people get the jobs and relationships they want. Perfect people love and like themselves, and they are liked and loved by others."

The **Guilt-Tripper** swoops in to criticize us for being wrong, not doing enough, or not *being* enough when we fall short of perfection or mess up. The Guilt-Tripper, much like the Perfectionist, wants to keep you safe and alive by keeping you well-behaved.

The **Control Freak** wants things to be predictable (or predictably chaotic in some cases!) and pushes itself and others to stay within these predictable states. Remember, the Control Freak is a part. It isn't your true self but is instead a defense mechanism developed to keep you safe.

The **Taskmaster** wants us to work, work hard, and work now. "Be more productive!" it tells us. It puts a lot of pressure on us to do things but also to do them the so-called "right" way. The Taskmaster tries to keep you safe and alive by making you a productive member of society.

The **Underminer** can be very deceptive, even seemingly kind. The Underminer tells us that we can't do something or that we'll never get a certain desired prize. "Don't try that; you won't be any good at it." "That sounds embarrassing; do something else instead." "Aim for a lower-paying job." "That person is out of your league." In this way, the Underminer convinces us that this *perspective* is actually reality.

The **Conformist** is another part that thinks there's a right and wrong way to be. The Conformist wants us to fit in by doing things "right." This part experiences anxiety, guilt, and shame around going against the grain. Like the Underminer, the Conformist tries to keep you safe and alive by limiting your visibility.

The **Destroyer** doesn't want us to exist. This is an especially difficult part to deal with. Suicidal thoughts and feelings are part of the Destroyer, and this is scary! The Destroyer urges us to give up, numb out, or even end our own lives as an escape from pain.

QUIZ: What kinds of Inner Critic parts do you have?

Mark the statements below that sound like what you do, say, or hear in your head when it comes to feeling critical of yourself and others. The key at the bottom of the list will tell you which parts correspond with each statement. It is, of course, possible to have all the archetypes of Inner Critics in your system of parts. For now, focus on recognizing which of these scenarios sound like your Critic habits. Answer "True" or "False" to the following:

1. I compare myself to others and wonder why I don't try harder to be like them.

2. I can get more people to like and appreciate me if I just fix myself.

3. I can do everything right if I try hard enough.

4. Sometimes I don't care if I live or die.

5. I wonder if life is really worth it to keep going.

6. I only feel okay when I'm asleep, intoxicated, or binge eating.

7. I hate when other people bring their issues into my personal space.

8. I hate when other people tell me I'm wrong.

9. I like showing others a better way to do things.

10. I can never have the kind of job I really want.

11. I'm afraid to try new activities. I would embarrass myself.

12. I only feel at peace when everything is going my way.

13. I feel terrible when I offend someone.

14. I still feel awful about things I did years ago.

15. I beat myself up for making mistakes.

16. My value in this world is determined by what I accomplish and contribute.

17. I should've done more in my life by now.

18. Happiness is for other people. I'm just satisfied to get by in life.

19. People judge me for not being more normal. I try to be normal, but I guess I'm a weirdo.

20. If I want to be happy and successful, I have to act a certain way.

21. I wish I could figure out what makes me different and then fix it.

KEY

If you answered "True" to any of the previous statements, it's likely you have the corresponding part listed below. There can be more overlap than just what's listed, so trust your own experience. You can use this quiz to better recognize, understand, and work with your Inner Critic parts.

1. Perfectionist or Taskmaster
2. Perfectionist or Conformist
3. Perfectionist or Taskmaster
4. Destroyer
5. Destroyer
6. Destroyer
7. Control Freak
8. Control Freak
9. Control Freak
10. Underminer
11. Underminer
12. Perfectionist
13. Guilt-Tripper
14. Guilt-Tripper
15. Guilt-Tripper
16. Taskmaster
17. Taskmaster
18. Underminer
19. Conformist
20. Conformist
21. Conformist

The Inner Critic Worksheet

These exercises will help you identify and work with your Inner Critic parts. Use these activities with the Critic quiz to help understand and discern specific Critic archetypes. For additional resources to help you with this work, visit https://RezoomBook.com. Get to know your Inner Critic:

1. Choose a familiar Inner Critic part. In your memory, go back to a time or specific moment when that part was active.

2. See if you can notice this part as a sensation in your body. If so, notice where it is and how it feels. Bring your awareness to this sensation.

3. Let an image form in your mind. What does this part look like? Where is it? Does it look like a person, a cartoon, or an object? Does the part have any other sensory qualities, like a smell, a sensation, or a sound?

4. Now imagine moving that part out of your body and away, so that it's some distance from you (e.g., six feet away, other side of the room). Notice how you feel toward this part. See if you can lean into being curious and open to this part and what it can teach you.

5. Ask the part how it's trying to help you. Don't think or analyze; just listen in and see how it responds. Ask the part, "What are you afraid will happen if you don't help me in this way?" Note the answer the part gives you.

6. Ask the part how old it thinks you are. If it thinks you're younger than you are, update the part so it knows how old you are now. Thank this part for its efforts to help you. Tell the part that you can do the job of protecting yourself from now on.

7. If you are able, thank this part for its positive intentions. Know that you've begun to develop a relationship with it. Now do some journaling to describe what you've learned about this part. You may also want to draw an image of it, give it a name, and take any other steps that will make the part more real and personal to you.

MORE ACTIVITIES

1. **Replace Critics with curiosity.** When you're unblended, you'll feel confident and curious about yourself and your parts. Inner Critics lead you away from this confidence and comfort in your own skin. They'll tell you you're bad or that you have to suffer or do without. When you feel these parts taking over and attempting to blend, take some deep breaths. Do a grounding meditation. Then get curious about what's happening in your mind, your external life, and your body.

2. **Identify the strategies used by your Critic parts.** What are all the ways these parts work to protect you and keep you the same? When did you notice the Critic parts showing up in your life?

3. **Write a story about what happens in your life— internal and external, personal and public—if a Critic part is healed and kept unblended.** How do the other parts react? Does the system fall apart, or do the other parts work overtime? Or is there another outcome entirely? Who would you be if you didn't hear this criticism in your head anymore?

THE ISOLATOR PARTS

The Isolator parts interfere with many qualities of a happy, authentic life, but the most glaring disruption is to our connection to a supportive community. Isolators may do this physically by avoiding actual contact or emotionally by being aloof, silent, or otherwise "unknowable." By withdrawing, this part protects us from others' judgment, intrusion, and violation of our boundaries. It is here to keep us safe: safe from judgment, safe from abuse, and safe from others, as well as ourselves.

One of the most common Isolators is the **Diminisher**. This part tells you that you're not important and that your needs aren't really worth others' time and attention. When you think about reaching out for help or connection, the Diminisher tells you such things as, "You should know how to deal with this on your own. Don't be a burden. No one is interested in your issues. This isn't that important."

The **Procrastinator** is a part that we can find in any situation, from work to love to physical health. "I'll do it tomorrow. Now is not a good time. What difference does it make if I do it tomorrow or next week?" When we are in this loop, we can avoid connecting with others forever.

The **Cynic** distrusts everyone: family, friends, strangers, even their God or higher power. The Cynic believes that everyone will ultimately disappoint it. This Isolator tells us that it's safer and happier to stay aloof and alone.

The **Soloist** believes that we do better alone. We can complete our goals better if no one else is holding us back with their needs or their methods of working. The Soloist usually judges others, but it works with Inner Critics that are very critical of us.

The **Workaholic** is one of those tricky Isolators that doesn't *seem* to be actively avoiding connection to others. The Workaholic has no time for social activities. This Isolator will tell us that we can't go have fun, see friends, or meet new people because there are tasks to finish: paid work, homework, chores, volunteer service, or other tasks.

The **Secret Keeper** is often intimately tied to shame. The Secret Keeper can keep us safe from shame and judgment by keeping behaviors or feelings secret. A Secret Keeper tends to work with the Oblivionator/Binger, and it's almost always present in addiction patterns.

The **Incognito** wants us to be invisible, especially in a crowd. It keeps us unknown, plain, and under the radar. The Incognito is especially common in individuals who fear romance, sexual contact, and other forms of emotional and physical intimacy. The Incognito is not the same as being asexual or aromantic; those are sexual orientations, while the Isolator parts are defense mechanisms to keep us hidden and anonymous.

The **Misfit** part says we simply don't belong. Most importantly, the Misfit *doesn't want to belong*. It wants to be isolated and safe. The Misfit is one of the Isolators that can use extroversion to push others away and remain unknowable. It can give us a feeling of power and control in making ourselves unapproachable.

The **One-Night Stander** is an extroverted part that can be sexually promiscuous, but it can manifest in other ways. This part uses flirting, sex, and other forms of intense interaction to avoid getting *emotionally* close to people. The One-Night Stander may have frequent sex or go to many parties, but no one really knows it.

The **Luddite** is an Isolator that tells us that we're not good with technology, or don't really understand email or texting or social media. Instead of being curious and open to learning new ways to connect to others, the Luddite says we'll never really understand how these modes of connection work.

The **Screen Addict** is the reverse of the Luddite, but the two can easily work together. The Screen Addict spends lots of time absorbed in screen time. Instead of connecting with others or sharing the experience of watching TV or playing a video game, the Screen Addict stays alone, absorbed in the technology and avoiding contact with others.

QUIZ: What kinds of Isolator parts do you have?

Which of these parts show up for you around closeness, vulnerability, and connection to others? Mark the statements below that sound like what you do, say, or hear in your head when it comes to interacting with or being seen by others. The key at the bottom of the list will tell you which parts correspond with each statement. It is, of course, possible to have all the archetypes of Isolators in your system of parts. For now, focus on recognizing which of these scenarios sound like your Isolator habits. Answer "True" or "False" to the following:

1. I don't want to be a burden on others.

2. My needs aren't that important.

3. I'm strong enough to handle this alone.

4. I should know how to do this by myself.

5. I don't like texting. People need to leave me alone.

6. I never know what to say in emails. I embarrass myself when I try to write them.

7. I'd much rather play games or use the Internet than talk to people.

8. I'm not really isolated. I text people or talk to them online, even if I don't go out and meet people in person.

9. I don't have time right now to ask for help.

10. It doesn't matter if I do this now or later.

11. This isn't a good time to be social or have conversations.

12. I can't really trust anyone.

13. Everyone disappoints me eventually.

14. I always end up driving people away.

15. I can't let anyone see how much I eat or what I do when I'm alone.

16. I can do whatever I want, as long as I don't get caught.

17. I don't want people staring at me. I don't want strangers to talk to me or flirt with me.

18. If I'm heavy, people won't be sexually attracted to me, and that's for the best.

19. I do my best work alone.

20. Others are too distracting; they're a liability when I'm trying to get things done.

21. I can't have a social life. I have work to do.

22. I get enough enjoyment from my projects. I don't need more friends.

23. People don't really "get" me, and that's fine. I'm just different.

24. Most people are boring and not worth my time.

25. Sex is so much easier than romance and relationships.

26. Being attractive and popular is preferable to being vulnerable.

KEY

If you answered "True" to any of the previous statements, it's likely you have the corresponding part listed below. There can be more overlap than just what's listed, so trust your own experience. You can use this quiz to better recognize, understand, and work with your Isolator parts.

1. Diminisher
2. Diminisher
3. Diminisher
4. Diminisher
5. Luddite
6. Luddite
7. Screen Addict
8. Screen Addict
9. Procrastinator
10. Procrastinator
11. Procrastinator
12. Cynic
13. Cynic
14. Secret Keeper
15. Secret Keeper
16. Secret Keeper
17. Incognito
18. Incognito
19. Soloist
20. Soloist
21. Workaholic
22. Workaholic
23. Misfit
24. Misfit
25. One-Night Stander
26. One-Night Stander

The Isolator Worksheet

These exercises will help you identify and work with your Isolator parts. Use these activities with the Isolator quiz to help understand and discern specific Isolator archetypes. For additional resources to help you with this work, visit https://RezoomBook.com. Get to know your Isolator:

1. Choose a familiar Isolator part. In your memory, go back to a time or specific moment when that part was active.

2. See if you can notice this part as a sensation in your body. If so, notice where it is and how it feels. Bring your awareness to this sensation.

3. Let an image form in your mind. What does this part look like? Where is it? Does it look like a person, a cartoon, or an object? Does the part have any other sensory qualities, like a smell, a sensation, or a sound?

4. Now imagine moving that part out of your body and away, so that it's some distance from you (e.g., six feet away, other side of the room). Notice how you feel toward this part. See if you can lean into being curious and open to this part and what it can teach you.

5. Ask the part how it's trying to help you. Don't think or analyze; just listen in and see how it responds. Ask the part, "What are you afraid will happen if you don't help me in this way?" Note the answer the part gives you.

6. Ask the part how old it thinks you are. If it thinks you're younger than you are, update the part so it knows how old you are now. Thank this part for its efforts to help you. Tell the part that you can do the job of protecting yourself from now on.

7. If you are able, thank this part for its positive intentions. Know that you've begun to develop a relationship with it. Now do some journaling to describe what you've learned about this Isolator part. You may also want to draw an image of it, give it a name, and take any other steps that will make the part more real and personal to you.

MORE ACTIVITIES

1. **Trade an Isolator for a connection.** When your Isolators want you to hide and become invisible, keep secrets, or otherwise avoid or reject other people, you can choose to pay attention. Community is one of the most important elements in healing parts and leaving old patterns behind. Your Isolators are protecting you from toxic, critical people, but once the Isolator is

unblended, you'll see how many people are neither toxic nor critical, especially in recovery communities full of people who are learning to identify and end these harmful behaviors.

2. **Make a connection map of all the people in your support network.** If the support is only one-sided (e.g., you're not giving any support back to the other party, or the other party isn't supporting you), make those connection lines a particular color or pattern, such as a dotted line. Go ahead and connect these individuals to each other as well if there are support connections among them. What do you notice about this map? How connected and supported are you compared to the others in your web?

3. **Write down what is lost when you isolate from them.** Not only do we lose out on connection and support when we isolate, but our friends and family also lose that support. Write out what you lose through isolation, and then write out what others lose when you're never around or available. Explore what happens when you hide from others.

4. **Identify the strategies used by your Isolator parts.** What are all the ways your Isolator parts work to protect you and keep you isolated? When did you notice the Isolator parts showing up in your life?

5. **Write a story about what happens in your life— internal and external, personal and public—if an Isolator part is healed and kept unblended.** How do the other parts react? Does the system fall apart, or do the other parts work overtime? Or is there another outcome entirely?

ENDNOTES

Chapter 2

1. *Susan Peirce Thompson, Bright Line Eating: The Science of Living Happy, Thin, and Free* (Carlsbad, CA: Hay House, 2017), 70.

2. Paul C. Fletcher and Paul J. Kenny, "Food Addiction: A Valid Concept?" *Neuropsychopharmacology* 43, no. 13 (December 2018): 2506–13; Eliza L. Gordon et al., "What Is the Evidence for 'Food Addiction'? A Systematic Review," *Nutrients* 10, no. 4 (April 2018): 477.

3. Ashley N. Gearhardt, Erica M. Schulte, and Emma T. Schiestl, "Food Addiction Prevalence: Development and Validation of Diagnostic Tools," in *Compulsive Eating Behavior and Food Addiction: Emerging Pathological Constructs*, ed. Pietro Cottone et al. (Cambridge, MA: Academic Press, 2019), 15–33.

4. *Yale News*, July 9, 2007.

5. Ibid.

6. American Psychiatric Association, *Diagnostic and Statistical Manual of Mental Disorders*, 5th Edition (*DSM-5*) (Washington, DC: American Psychiatric Publishing, 2013), 481.

7. Ibid., 483–484.

8. Marketdata LLC, "The U.S. Weight Loss & Diet Control Market," Marketresearch.com, 2018.

9. Centers for Disease Control and Prevention, National Center for Health Statistics, "Underlying Cause of Death, 1999–2019," on CDC WONDER Online Database. Vital Statistics Cooperative Program, 2020.

10. American Psychiatric Association, *Diagnostic and Statistical Manual of Mental Disorders*, 5th Edition (*DSM-5*) (Washington, DC: American Psychiatric Publishing, 2013), 483.

11. Centers for Disease Control and Prevention, *National Diabetes Statistics Report, 2020* (Atlanta, GA: Centers for Disease Control and Prevention, U.S. Dept of Health and Human Services, 2020).

12. Yuki Izumi et al., "Risk of Reamputation in Diabetic Patients Stratified by Limb and Level of Amputation: A 10-Year Observation," *Diabetes Care* 29, no. 3 (March 2006): 566–70.

13. Gordon et al., "What Is the Evidence for 'Food Addiction'?"

14. Emilie Lacroix and Kristin M. von Ranson, "Prevalence of Social, Cognitive, and Emotional Impairment among Individuals with Food Addiction,"

Eating and Weight Disorders—Studies on Anorexia, Bulimia and Obesity (26, no. 4 (May 2021): 1253-58.

15. Christopher Rodrigue, Sylvain Iceta, and Catherine Bégin, "Food Addiction and Cognitive Functioning: What Happens in Adolescents?" *Nutrients* 12, no. 12 (November 2020): 3633.

16. Joan Ifland, Marianne T. Marcus, and Harry G. Preuss, *Processed Food Addiction: Foundations, Assessment, and Recovery* (Boca Raton, FL: CRC Press, 2018), 6.

Chapter 3

17. Nikolaas Tinbergen, *The Study of Instinct* (Oxford, UK: Clarendon Press, 1989).

18. Antonio Stasi et al., "Neuromarketing Empirical Approaches and Food Choice: A Systematic Review," *Food Research International* 108 (June 2018): 650–64.

Chapter 5

19. David G. Blanchflower, Andrew J. Oswald, and Sarah Stewart-Brown, "Is Psychological Well-Being Linked to the Consumption of Fruit and Vegetables?" *Social Indicators Research* 114, no. 3 (October 2012): 785–801.

20. Bonnie A. White, Caroline C. Horwath, and Tamlin S. Conner, "Many Apples a Day Keep the Blues Away—Daily Experiences of Negative and Positive Affect and Food Consumption in Young Adults," *British Journal of Health Psychology* 18, no. 4 (November 2013): 782–98.

21. Daniel J. Simons and Daniel T. Levin, "Change Blindness," *Trends in Cognitive Sciences* 1, no. 7 (October 1997): 261–67.

22. Daniel J. Simons and Christopher F. Chabris, "Gorillas in Our Midst: Sustained Inattentional Blindness for Dynamic Events," *Perception* 28, no. 9 (September 1999): 1059–74.

23. Daniel J. Simons, "Attentional Capture and Inattentional Blindness," *Trends in Cognitive Sciences* 4, no. 4 (April 2000): 147–55.

Chapter 6

24. Antoine Lutz et al., "Long-Term Meditators Self-Induce High-Amplitude Gamma Synchrony during Mental Practice," *Proceedings of the National Academy of Sciences* 101, no. 46 (November 2004): 16369–73.

25. Martin Seligman, "Find Three Good Things Each Day," *Action for Happiness*, http://www.actionforhappiness.org/take-action/find-three-good-things-each-day.

26. Maud Purcell, "The Health Benefits of Journaling," *Psych Central*, May 17, 2016, https://psychcentral.com/lib/the-health-benefits-of-journaling#1.

27. A. E. Kazdin, "Reactive Self-Monitoring: The Effects of Response Desirability, Goal Setting, and Feedback," *Journal of Consulting and Clinical Psychology* 42, no. 5 (October 1974): 704–16, doi:10.1037/h0037050.

28. Stephan J. Guyenet, *The Hungry Brain: Outsmarting the Instincts That Make Us Overeat* (New York: Flatiron Books, 2017), 269.

Chapter 7

29. James S. House, Karl R. Landis, and Debra Umberson, "Social Relationships and Health," *Science* 241, no. 4865 (July 1988): 540–45.

30. Michael Kosfeld et al., "Oxytocin Increases Trust in Humans," *Nature* 435, no. 7042 (June 2005): 673–76.

31. Bethany E. Kok et al., "How Positive Emotions Build Physical Health: Perceived Positive Social Connections Account for the Upward Spiral between Positive Emotions and Vagal Tone," *Psychological Science* 24, no. 7 (May 2013): 1123–32.

32. Steve W. Cole et al., "Social Regulation of Gene Expression in Human Leukocytes," *Genome Biology* 8, no. 9 (September 2007): 1–13.

33. Ed Diener and Martin E.P. Seligman, "Very Happy People," *Psychological Science* 13, no. 1 (January 2002): 81–84.

34. Lucy E. Keniger et al., "What Are the Benefits of Interacting with Nature?" *International Journal of Environmental Research and Public Health* 10, no. 3 (March 2013): 913–35.

INDEX

A

abstinence
  from flour and sugar, 1
  perfectionism and, 51–55
  as squeaky clean Bright Lines, 6
accountability
  Accountability Calls (phone call experiment), 106, 147–150
  accountability tolerance, 168–169
  looking backward for, 120–123
actions, 97–135
  automaticity with, 97–99
  committing to process for, 102–103
  as daily rituals, 105–106
  defined, 97
  evening routine for, 118–134 (*see also* evening routine)
  feelings, thoughts, and, 103–105
  getting started with, 131
  as habit stack, 106–108, 119
  identity and, 99–101
  Inner Critic Part for, 136–137
  morning routine for, 108–118 (*see also* morning routine)
activities, giving up/reducing (Substance Use Disorder criteria), 31
AIR (automaticity, identity, rezoom), 165–167
alcohol, 77–78
alone time, 159–160
American Psychiatric Association, 27–33
amygdala, 60–61, 113
anorexia nervosa, 26
artificial sweeteners, 9
Atomic Habits (Clear), 99–101, 127–128

Authentic Self. *see also* Parts Work
  control vs. spontaneity, 48
  8 Cs (calm, confidence, curiosity, creativity, clarity, courage, compassion, connectedness), 18–19, 76
  Food Indulger and, 37
  life-changing shifts for, 56–57 (*see also* Rezoom System)
  tuning in to, 74–78
automaticity
  with actions, 97–99
  AIR (automaticity, identity, rezoom), 165–167
  importance of, 83–85
  of room-by-room habit stack, 119
  support and, 160–162
awareness, 12, 87–88

B

Barks, Coleman, 124
basal ganglia, 58–59
Baumeister, Roy F., 51
bed, making, 111
behavioral addictions, 41
behavior change (actions, feelings, thoughts), 103–105. *see also* actions
Bem, Daryl, 102–103
BFF (Breathe, Feel your body, Find your Feet), 115
binge eating disorder, 82
brain. *see also* hormones
  addiction and effect on, 41–47
  amygdala and fight-or-flight, 113–114
  basal ganglia, 58–59
  fear and panic by, 60–61
  Food Controller Parts Work for, 48–50

ACKNOWLEDGMENTS

FROM THE DESK (AND HEART) OF
SUSAN PEIRCE THOMPSON

It's hard to describe the horror of starting this amazing worldwide movement, only to watch myself fall into the ditch with my own food and then struggle for years to stay consecutively Bright. And now, having been Bright for a lovely stretch of time, supported every day by the Rezoom Reframe, I sit in the truism that our deepest pain and most pernicious struggles can pave the way for meaningful service to others if we humble ourselves and watch for the lessons. If I hadn't gone through those breaks, over and over, this book wouldn't have been possible. It's a gift born of pain—and the grace of unstoppability.

With that knowledge, I am overwhelmed with gratitude for the people who supported me during that time. Especially my Mastermind Mavens: Cathy Cox, Linden Morris Delrio, and Marianne Marsh. My beloved Christine (Chris) Gimeno Davis. Diane O'Haron. Gabe Enz, Georgia Whitney, and Lou Capuano. Sage Lavine and Ocean Robbins. Dana Oliver, Anne Wax, Patricia O'Connor, Penny Gibson, and Stacey Carpenter. You were all there for me when I felt beyond aid. Thank you for lighting a candle and sitting with me in the cave.

The incomparable BLE Team. When I came out of the cave and brought the Rezoom Reframe to you in 2018, you marshaled the infrastructure to create the course that very December and we started changing lives with this approach. You are so bright, so committed, so hardworking, so fun. So open and honest. I am outrageously lucky to work with you every day, and you bless me in more ways than I can ever express. Thank you for all that you do—for me, and for this movement.

To the Bright Lifers and all the folks in BLE Land who took Reboot Rezoom, offered feedback, wrote in to customer support, shared comments, watched videos, and committed wholeheartedly to their Bright Transformations. To those who demonstrate every day in ways big and small the awe-inspiring perseverance of living the reframe. Serving you is my life's work.

My unparalleled videographer, Daniel Maggio of Fish Tank Video. Reboot Rezoom was created with your nonstop support—thank you, always.

My co-author, Everett Considine. I love you and am so grateful to be on this journey with you. Your innovative and powerful application of Parts Work has helped me know what my system really needs when it's telling me it needs to eat. Thank you for your brilliance and insight working with countless Bright Lifers, for seeing the big important patterns, and for contributing your wisdom as I evolved the course into this book.

None of my books would have found their way into the world without my gracious agent, Lucinda Blumenfeld. How is it possible that such a talented agent could be simultaneously such a fierce advocate and so very much fun to work with? I pinch myself.

Once again, it's been incredible to work with the team at Hay House. Reid Tracy, Patty Gift, and Sally Mason-Swaab, it's such a pleasure and a gift to be a Hay House author. Thank you for going above and beyond for me, these past couple of years especially. You are like no publishing team on earth. Lisa Cheng, you are the most extraordinary editor, and I am so grateful for your insight and skill. You elevated this book with every draft.

Ashley Bernardi and the amazing team at Nardi Media, you are my heart's delight, and every time I have a catch-up call with you on my calendar, I just squeal. Thank you for everything you do to help grow the movement and spread the word.

Win Guan, you tracked down countless references and then went to find yet more. I gave you so little to work with, and you always came through. I am grateful for your willingness, availability, and scientific precision.

My fabulous proofreaders for their steady eye and keen insight: Sharon Cheek, Jackie Montarra, and Sunny St. Pierre; and Eileen Lass of The Lass Word Proofreading and Editing.

Nicola Wheir, you know this book is yours. Our third together and I just cannot imagine a better soul sister to write with. You held the torch for this book from the very beginning when I had too much on my plate. Thank you for believing wholeheartedly in the potential of this book until I could come around. I am so grateful for your wit and friendship, your wisdom and patience.

Tayler Thomson and Claire Lobban, thank you for being splendid and matchless as you keep the Thompson household running and my inbox managed. I treasure each of you so much. None of it would work without you.

Gary Wolk, thank you for helping me navigate the ethics of a case study.

Mom, you will always have my gratitude for decades of deep maternal care. I was not an easy kid to raise, and your love was a constant.

And to my dad, thank you for being the best cheerleader; I love you with all my heart. (And can we all please look as spectacular as you at 80? Possibly? Yes??)

My beloved husband, David. We went through a lot over the course of writing this book and emerged stronger, more dedicated, and more in love than ever. Thank you for standing by me through all my ups and downs with food and supporting me in keeping my Lines Bright, always. Our partnership is exquisite and so well-balanced. I love you.

And finally, my girls, Zoe, Robin, and Maya, thank you for your support and encouragement. Being your mom is such a precious gift. A friend of mine recently said, "Here's the thing about parenting. Around age twelve, you get fired as their manager, and then you have to work really hard to get hired back as their consultant." I pray every day to earn a place by your side. I love you more than I can ever express.

• • •

FROM THE DESK (AND HEART)
OF EVERETT CONSIDINE

I feel so blessed to be doing work that I love that is having such an 0.important impact on the world. The ideas presented in this book are the distillation of about 10 years of working with Internal Family Systems and 6 years of working with Bright Line Eating. I'd like to thank those who have supported me along the way and those who continue to do so.

First off, my deepest thanks to Char Sundust. You are an incredible mentor and teacher. It was your support and unconditional belief in me that allowed me to transition from the world of technology to the world of healing and teaching. You continue to be the model for me of what a spiritual teacher should be. Thanks for showing me what it looks like to have power and integrity.

And deep thanks to Dina Love. Thank you, Soul Sister. It was you who introduced me to IFS. You somehow saw how perfect it was for me. I so value your presence in my life. I've always felt seen by you. Thanks for continuing to show me what's next. You continue to inspire me and to put the wind into my sails.

Thanks to Dick Schwartz, the creator of IFS. Words can't express the gratitude I feel toward you. Thank you for the insight to open this training to those outside of traditional therapist roles. You are such a worthy steward of this powerful healing modality.

Thanks to Jay Earley. Our friendship is so important to me. Much of my content in this book was modeled on a style of Parts Work that I learned from you. You continue to inspire me professionally and personally.

Thanks to Bonnie Weiss. You were talking about the Indulger/ Controller Polarization long before me. Thanks for inspiring me as I evolved my approach to IFS and eating issues.

Thanks to Evan Peterson. Wow, our journey together has been amazing. So much of your beautiful writing has become part of my teachings. You are such a brilliant and clever writer. It feels so good to be able to lean on you.

Deepest thanks to Susan Peirce Thompson, my co-author and friend. You inspire me beyond measure. Thank you for seeing me. Thank you for giving me free rein. Your trust in me allowed the deepest levels of creativity to open for me. Being on this journey with you has truly been a magic carpet ride. I can't wait to see what is ahead of us.

Thanks to Trevor Slocum. You are so special to me. Thanks for being such an incredible witness and friend. Your support has allowed me to do more and be more. I know, because of you, I am a better man.

Thanks to Nicola Wheir. Your ability to move forward and get things done is awe-inspiring. You've made the process of writing this book feel both fun and safe. I'm so grateful Susan brought us together.

Thanks to Tara Bogdon. You are my behind-the-scenes partner in crime at BLE. Thank you for always being available even at the weirdest hours. Thanks for keeping me on track and always making sure I have a deadline to inspire me. We've been together on this whole ride!

Thanks to Patricia O'Conner. You were the sponsor I needed when I was struggling with my Finish Line Anxiety. Your support and sage counsel help so many. Thanks for teaching me about the recovery mindset.

Thanks to Zoe Nicholson. I love you. Thanks for inspiring me in so many ways. You've been writing books for years. Your writing inspired me to write. Look what happened!

Thanks to Zoe Alexander and the Maui Forum. You brought me to Maui to teach! Those classes formed the basis of what was to come. Thank you for inviting us to Maui so that we could make it our home.

Thanks to my mom and dad, Linda Gentry and Rett Considine. If you were still here, Mom, I know you'd be so proud of me. I know that you are, Dad.

Thanks to Karen, my sister, and her beautiful family. It's just us now! I'm always here for you.

And finally, deepest thanks to my husband, Sam Garcia. You truly are the light of my life. You are my spiritual life partner and soul mate. Your beautiful presence in my life allows me to fly even higher. Your dedication to your spiritual practice and emotional healing is a continuous source of inspiration for me. Thanks for wanting me. Your love has healed me in so many ways.

ABOUT THE AUTHORS

SUSAN PEIRCE THOMPSON, PH.D., is the *New York Times* best-selling author of *Bright Line Eating* and *The Official Bright Line Eating Cookbook*. She is an adjunct associate professor of brain and cognitive sciences at the University of Rochester and an expert in the psychology of eating. She is president of the Institute for Sustainable Weight Loss and the founder and CEO of Bright Line Eating Solutions, a company dedicated to helping people achieve long-term, sustainable weight loss. She lives in Rochester, New York, with her husband, David, and their three daughters. You can visit her online at BrightLineEating.com.

EVERETT CONSIDINE is a certified Internal Family Systems practitioner and transformational coach. He is the creator and teacher of Bright Line Freedom, Bright Line Eating's Parts Work course. He has trained and coached thousands of Bright Lifers and helped them settle peacefully into the program. He has a deep background in meditation and Eastern spirituality and loves introducing people to Internal Family Systems. He lives in Maui, Hawaii, with his husband, Sam Garcia, where they host transformational retreats and see coaching clients remotely. You can find him online at EverettConsidine.com.

Hay House Titles of Related Interest

We hope you enjoyed this Hay House book. If you'd like to receive our online catalog featuring additional information on Hay House books and products, or if you'd like to find out more about the Hay Foundation, please contact:

Hay House, Inc., P.O. Box 5100, Carlsbad, CA 92018-5100
(760) 431-7695 or (800) 654-5126
(760) 431-6948 (fax) or (800) 650-5115 (fax)
www.hayhouse.com® • www.hayfoundation.org

———

Published in Australia by: Hay House Australia Pty. Ltd.,
18/36 Ralph St., Alexandria NSW 2015
Phone: 612-9669-4299 • *Fax:* 612-9669-4144
www.hayhouse.com.au

Published in the United Kingdom by: Hay House UK, Ltd.,
The Sixth Floor, Watson House, 54 Baker Street, London W1U 7BU
Phone: +44 (0)20 3927 7290 • *Fax:* +44 (0)20 3927 7291
www.hayhouse.co.uk

Published in India by: Hay House Publishers India,
Muskaan Complex, Plot No. 3, B-2, Vasant Kunj, New Delhi 110 070
Phone: 91-11-4176-1620 • *Fax:* 91-11-4176-1630
www.hayhouse.co.in

———

Access New Knowledge.
Anytime. Anywhere.

Learn and evolve at your own pace
with the world's leading experts.

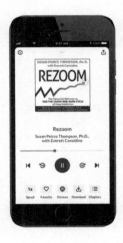